Current Topics in
Environmental Health and Preventive Medicine

Series editor

T. Otsuki
Kurashiki, Japan

Current Topics in Environmental Health and Preventive Medicine, published in partnership with the Japanese Society of Hygiene, is designed to deliver well written volumes authored by experts from around the globe, covering the prevention and environmental health related to medical, biological, molecular biological, genetic, physical, psychosocial, chemical, and other environmental factors. The series will be a valuable resource to both new and established researchers, as well as students who are seeking comprehensive information on environmental health and health promotion.

More information about this series at http://www.springer.com/series/13556

Takemi Otsuki • Claudia Petrarca
Mario Di Gioacchino

Editors

Allergy and Immunotoxicology in Occupational Health

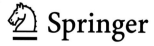 Springer

Editors
Takemi Otsuki
Department of Hygiene
Kawasaki Medical School
Kurashiki, Japan

Mario Di Gioacchino
Immuntotoxicology and Allergy Unit &
  Occupational Biorepository, Center of
  Excellence on Aging and
  Translational Medicine (CeSI-MeT)
"G. D'Annunzio" University Foundation
Chieti, Italy

Department of Medicine and Science
  of Aging
G. d'Annunzio University
Chieti, Italy

Claudia Petrarca
Immuntotoxicology and Allergy Unit &
  Occupational Biorepository, Center of
  Excellence on Aging and Translational
  Medicine (CeSI-MeT)
"G. D'Annunzio" University Foundation
Chieti, Italy

ISSN 2364-8333   ISSN 2364-8341   (electronic)
Current Topics in Environmental Health and Preventive Medicine
ISBN 978-981-10-0349-3   ISBN 978-981-10-0351-6   (eBook)
DOI 10.1007/978-981-10-0351-6

Library of Congress Control Number: 2016953187

Printed on acid-free paper

This Springer imprint is published by Springer Nature
The registered company is Springer Science+Business Media Singapore Pte Ltd.

Preface

This Book is published as a mid-term step (i.e., middle of every 3-year period) by the Allergy and Immunotoxicology Scientific Committee (AISC) of the International Congress of Occupational Health (ICOH). The comprehensive meeting of ICOH is held every 3 years. Recently, it was held in Seoul, South Korea, 31 May–5 June 2015, when Prof. Mario Di Gioacchino, of Chieti, Italy, served as the chairperson. The next meeting will be held in Dublin, Ireland, in 2018. In conjunction with the opening of the special, general, oral, and poster sessions as well as joint sessions with other scientific committees (SCs), several SCs are staging mid-term activities independently. Our SC/AISC has also been holding several special midterm symposiums in Italy, China, and Japan (in Kumamoto and Kyoto) and calls each such symposium an *International Symposium on Occupational and Environmental Allergy and Immune Diseases* (ISOEAID). As the current chairperson of this SC, Prof. Otsuki was the local organizer of ISOEAID 2010 held at Kyoto. It was April and we were surrounded by beautiful cherry blossom trees in full bloom. During the symposium, we presented and discussed many issues regarding the occupational and environmental allergy and immunotoxicology field and enjoyed the lectures on air pollution such as the effects of PM2.5 on immune organs, immunological aspects of sick-building syndrome, sensitizers in GHS (The Globally Harmonized System of Classification and Labelling of Chemicals), and childhood and immunology.

The first honorary chairperson in our SCs was Prof. Toshio Matsushita, Kagoshima, Japan. Thereafter, Prof. Poalo Boscolo, Chieti, Italy, and Prof. Kanehisa Morimoto, Osaka, Japan, inherited the chairperson's role. All three editors of this eBook have been in that role in our SC. Prof. Di Gioacchino served as Chair 2009–2014. I have been the Chair since 2015, with Prof. Petrarca as the secretary in the SCs. Subsequently we decided to publish this eBook instead of ISOEAID at this mid-term point based on the presentation in the ICOH meeting in Seoul, South Korea.

The AISC has been focusing on investigation and discussion of the pathophysiological mechanisms involved with the allergic and immunotoxicological effects of environmental as well as occupational substances. Particularly, occupational allergies such as dermatitis and asthma were practically classical occupational diseases. The basic strategy is to avoid exposure, whereas there have been numerous newly developed substances that are being introduced in occupational situations. Thus, establishing methods of prediction using in vitro and *in silico* procedures is required. In addition to these investigations, epidemiological studies are also important, as is establishing a system to quickly identify allergic diseases caused by newer substances, and it is valuable, as well, to prevent workers from contracting these diseases. In addition, with allergic diseases the immunotoxicological effects of various substances in the environment as well as occupational settings are also important. Major members of our SC have been investigating the immunotoxicological effects of fibrous and particulate matters such as silica, asbestos, and recently nanomaterials including nanoparticles, nanotubes, and nanosheets.

In the specialty session for allergy, the review of prevention and management of allergens in occupational allergy, traditional and emerging occupational allergy in Japan, review of work-related and non-industrial indoor-related asthma, and molecular and cellular mechanisms in lung-specific immune responses activated by some particulates were presented. Regarding immunotoxicology, epidemiological health surveillance in formerly asbestos-exposed workers as well as experimental work regarding the effects of asbestos on human regulatory T cells were presented. In addition, understanding immunotoxicity of engineered nanomaterials for sustainable nanotechnology was also presented.

There were many poster presentations in Korea on glass allergic asthma, sensitization in workers exposed to urban air pollution, in silico analysis such as the qualitative structure–toxicity relationship (QSTR), solar radiation and the immune system, and phagocytic alteration in leukocytes exposed to benzene were the field I allergic insights. From the immunotoxicological aspect, many presentations regarding effects of asbestos on various human immune cells such as cytotoxic T cells (CTL), regulatory T cells as well as analysis of cytokines derived from asbestos-exposed patients such as pleural plaque and mesothelioma were discussed. As well, immunological alteration in silicosis patients who had been exposed to silica particles, induction of autoantibody production caused by mineral oil, and cell-cycle alteration in human peripheral lymphocytes exposed by palladium nanoparticles were presented. All the studies were very interesting and important to consider in further proceedings in prevention and management of occupational allergy and immunotoxicity.

The Allergy and Immunotoxicology SC has actively worked for understanding the pathophysiology of occupational allergy and immunotoxicity, prevention, and management of occupational environments as well as patients who have suffered from these pathological situations. In addition, we should participate in collaborative discussions, having scientific sessions with other SCs in ICOH, such as the Respiratory Disorders SC; Rural Health: Agriculture, Pesticides, and Organic Dust SC; Indoor Air Quality and Health SC; Occupational and Environmental Dermatoses SC; Occupational Toxicology SC; and others. Anyone involved with these SCs, please do not hesitate to contact our chairperson or secretary by e-mail. Let us aim for a good session at the Dublin meeting.

We welcome newcomers to our SC. Anyone who is interested in allergy and immunotoxicology issues, please contact us as soon as possible and let us support patients with these problems. We can contribute to the future construction of better occupational health management, especially with regard to allergy and immunotoxicology.

Kurashiki, Japan   Takemi Otsuki
Chiet, Italy   Mario Di Gioacchino
Chiet, Italy   Claudia Petrarca

Contents

1 **Suppressive Effects of Asbestos Exposure on the Human Immune Surveillance System**. 1
Yasumitsu Nishimura, Naoko Kumagai-Takei, Megumi Maeda,
Hidenori Matsuzaki, Suni Lee, Shoko Yamamoto, Tamayo Hatayama,
Kei Yoshitome, and Takemi Otsuki

2 **Silica-Induced Immunotoxicity: Chronic and Aberrant Activation of Immune Cells**. 15
Suni Lee, Hiroaki Hayashi, Hidenori Matsuzaki,
Naoko Kumagai-Takei, Megumi Maeda, Kei Yoshitome,
Shoko Yamamoto, Tamayo Hatayama, Yasumitsu Nishimura,
and Takemi Otsuki

3 **Engineered Nanomaterials and Occupational Allergy** 27
Claudia Petrarca, Luca Di Giampaolo, Paola Pedata,
Sara Cortese, and Mario Di Gioacchino

4 **Allergens in Occupational Allergy: Prevention and Management – Focus on Asthma**. 47
Mario Di Gioacchino, Luca Di Giampaolo, Veronica D'Ambrosio,
Federica Martino, Sara Cortese, Alessia Gatta, Loredana Della Valle,
Anila Farinelli, Rocco Mangifesta, Francesco Cipollone, Qiao Niu,
and Claudia Petrarca

5 **Particulate-Driven Type-2 Immunity and Allergic Responses**. 63
Etsushi Kuroda, Burcu Temizoz, Cevayir Coban,
Koji Ozasa, and Ken J. Ishii

6 **Traditional and Emerging Occupational Asthma in Japan** 83
Kunio Dobashi

**7   Skin Sensitization Model Based on Only Animal
Data by Qualitative Structure-Toxicity Relationships
(QSTR) Approach** 93
Kazuhiro Sato, Kohtaro Yuta, and Yukinori Kusaka

8   Non-industrial Indoor Environments and Work-Related Asthma... 103
Nicola Murgia, Ilenia Folletti, Giulia Paolocci,
Marco dell'Omo, and Giacomo Muzi

**9   Combined Effect on Immune and Nervous System
of Aluminum Nanoparticles** 115
Qiao Niu and Qinli Zhang

10 Non Pulmonary Effects of Isocyanates 129
Paola Pedata, Anna Rita Corvino, Monica Lamberti,
Claudia Petrarca, Luca Di Giampaolo, Nicola Sannolo,
and Mario Di Gioacchino

**11 Skin Exposure to Nanoparticles and Possible
Sensitization Risk** 143
Francesca Larese Filon

Chapter 1
Suppressive Effects of Asbestos Exposure on the Human Immune Surveillance System

Yasumitsu Nishimura, Naoko Kumagai-Takei, Megumi Maeda, Hidenori Matsuzaki, Suni Lee, Shoko Yamamoto, Tamayo Hatayama, Kei Yoshitome, and Takemi Otsuki

Abstract Asbestos exposure causes malignancies such as mesothelioma and lung cancer. Asbestos induces carcinogenic activity, and its fibers may cause immune-modifying effects that impair the immune surveillance system in regard to cancer cell monitoring. Impairment of natural killer (NK) cells, cytotoxic T lymphocytes (CTLs), T helper 1 (Th1) cells, and regulatory T (Treg) cells was investigated using cell lines and freshly isolated peripheral blood immune cells derived from health donors, as well as peripheral immune cells from asbestos-exposed patients with pleural plaque and malignant mesothelioma (MM). All findings showed that asbestos exposure caused reduction of antitumor immunity. Therefore, the carcinogenic and immune-modifying effects indicate that the immune surveillance system in relation to cancerous cells may be impaired by asbestos exposure.

Keywords Asbestos • NK cell • CTL • Th1 cell • Treg • Immune surveillance

Y. Nishimura • N. Kumagai-Takei • H. Matsuzaki • S. Lee • S. Yamamoto • T. Hatayama
K. Yoshitome • T. Otsuki (✉)
Department of Hygiene, Kawasaki Medical School,
577 Matsushima, Kurashiki, Okayama 701-0192, Japan
e-mail: takemi@med.kawasaki-m.ac.jp

M. Maeda
Department of Biofunctional Chemistry, Division of Bioscience, Okayama University
Graduate School of Natural Science and Technology,
1-1-1 Tsushima-Naka, Kita-Ku, Okayama 7008530, Japan

© Springer Science+Business Media Singapore 2017
T. Otsuki et al. (eds.), *Allergy and Immunotoxicology in Occupational Health*,
Current Topics in Environmental Health and Preventive Medicine,
DOI 10.1007/978-981-10-0351-6_1

1.1 Asbestos, Malignant Mesothelioma (MM), and Immune Function

Asbestos fibers have been used in many industrial fields worldwide because they are a natural mineral exhibiting high flexibility; resistance against heat, fire, friction, acids, and alkalis; as well as high electrical conductivity with a relatively low price for supply [1–4]. However, the majority of advanced nations have banned the use of asbestos due to its carcinogenicity (International Agency for Research on Cancer; IARC categorized asbestos as a definitive carcinogen in group 1), especially its association with lung cancer and MM, although many developing countries continue to use asbestos and several countries are currently exporting this mineral [5–8].

MM is a malignant tumor occurring in mesothelial cells located in the pleura, peritoneum, testicular serosa, and pericardium [9–11]. The major cause of MM is considered exposure to asbestos, with scant cases involving exposure to uranium and erionite (the frequent occurrence of MM in Cappadocia, Turkey, one of world's heritage sites, is known to be caused by erionite) [12–15]. It should be noted that MM in individuals exposed to asbestos results from relatively low to middle doses of exposure, compared with asbestosis/asbestos-induced lung fibrosis, a type of pneumoconiosis, which patients acquire after having been exposed to relatively high doses (according to the asbestos fibers found in the lung, i.e., more than two million fibers in 1 g dry lung tissue). In addition, the latent period is estimated as 30–50 years from the initial exposure to asbestos [9–11].

The carcinogenic actions of asbestos fibers are thought to be due to (1) oxygen stress, (2) chromosome tangling, and (3) absorption of other carcinogens in the lung. Considering these processes, crocidolite is thought to possess the strongest carcinogenic activity because it possesses the highest content of iron [16–20]. In addition, among the various asbestos fibers, the amphibole group, which includes crocidolite and amosite, is considered to have a stronger carcinogenic activity than the serpentine group, which only includes chrysotile, because of its physiological peculiarities and rigid form, and these considerations provide a basis for the above-mentioned carcinogenic hypotheses [16–20].

However, if we consider the long latent period, there may be biological effects of asbestos that cause malignancies other than the direct actions on alveolar and meso-thelial cells. An insight may be gained by considering the immunological effect because asbestos fibers are found in various lymph nodes and mainly in pulmonary regions, not only in asbestos-handling workers, but also in individuals exposed from the environment. In particular, investigation of individuals experiencing non-work-related exposure revealed higher asbestos contents in lymph nodes rather than the lung [21, 22]. The overall findings suggest a frequent association between asbestos fibers and immune cells, and recurrent and continuous exposure to asbestos may alter the cellular, molecular, and functional features of immune cells. A consideration of malignant tumors in asbestos-exposed people indicates that the immune effects of asbestos may comprise a reduced tumor immunity that makes individuals more prone to cancers after a long latent period.

1.2 Alteration of Various Immune Cells Caused by Asbestos Exposure

1.2.1 Natural Killer (NK) Cell

1.2.1.1 Human NK Cell Line, YT-A1

A human NK cell line, YT-A1, was cocultured continuously with 5 μg/ml of chrysotile B (CB) for more than 5 months (YT-CB5). The aforementioned concentration of CB was chosen for these experiments because it did not induce apoptosis or growth inhibition. Meanwhile, the cytotoxicity against K562, a human erythroleukemia cell line, and cell surface expression of various receptors were compared with those of the YT-A1 original cell line, which was never exposed to asbestos. After 5 months of cultivation, YT-CB5 showed decreased cytotoxicity with reduced expression of NK cell-activating receptors such as NKG2D and 2B4, whereas other surface markers such as CD16, NKG2A, and CD94 were not changed. Although killing of K562 cells is not dependent on the 2B4 receptor, YT-CB5 showed impairment of 2B4-dependent cytotoxicity as analyzed by a reverse antibody-dependent cellular cytotoxicity (ADCC) assay using the anti-2B4 antibody. In addition, YT-CB5 showed decreased phosphorylation of extracellular signal-regulated kinase (ERK) 1/2 after cultivation with K562 and stimulation with anti-NKG2D antibody. These results indicate that exposure to asbestos causes a reduction of NK cell cytotoxicity and decreased expression in activating receptors [23–28].

1.2.1.2 NK Cell Cytotoxicity in MM Patients

We investigated the state of NK cell cytotoxicity in patients with MM who might have been exposed to asbestos through the presence or absence of an occupational history with the mineral. After adjusting peripheral blood mononuclear cells (PBMC) from MM patients, cytotoxicity against K562 cells caused by 5,000 NK cells in PBMC and expression of NK cell-activating receptors were compared with those from healthy donors (HDs). NK cells derived from MM patients showed reduced cytotoxicity when compared with those from HD. Interestingly, although surface expression of NKG2D and 2B4 on NK cells from MM did not alter, another activating receptor, NKp46, exhibited reduced expression [23]. In response to this finding, we analyzed the expression of activating receptors on NK cells derived from HD and stimulated by interleukin (IL)-2 in vitro with or without 5 μg/ml of CB. Similar to NK cells from MM patients, there was a remarkable decrease in NKp46 expression, whereas expression of NKG2D and 2B4 did not decrease. In addition, the control substance used for CB, glass wool, did not induce these changes of expression of activating receptors. Thus, asbestos exposure specifically reduced the expression of NKp46 and resulted in reduced function of NK cells [23–28].

1.2.1.3   Relationship Between Killing Activity and Receptor Expressions

The relationship between expression levels of NK cell-activating receptors with the degree of cytotoxicity in HD and strength of downstream signaling receptors was examined. The killing activity against K562, expression levels of activating receptors, and phosphorylation levels of ERK 1/2 in NK cells derived from HD were measured. HDs whose NK cells revealed stronger killing activity showed higher expression of NKG2D and NKp46, as well as strong phosphorylation levels of ERK 1/2 molecules, when NK cells were simulated by anti-NKG2D or anti-NKp46 antibodies. However, killing activity was not correlated with expression levels of 2B4 or phosphorylation levels of ERK 1/2 in NK cells after stimulation by anti-2B4 antibody. The overall results showed that surface expression levels of NKG2D and NKp46 were important for cytotoxic activity in NK cells derived from asbestos-exposed patients. The overall results showed that the impairment of NK cells in these patients may be caused by decreased expression of these molecules induced by the continuous and recurrent exposure to asbestos [23–28].

1.2.2   Cytotoxic T Lymphocyte (CTL)

1.2.2.1   CTL Differentiation and Proliferation in Mixed Lymphocyte Reaction (MLR)

The MLR assay was used to evaluate CTL function derived from naïve CD8+ T cells cultured with allo-PBMC or splenic cells in vitro. Thus, to examine the effects of CB on CTL function, PBMC derived from HD were utilized for MLR using allo-PBMC with or without 5 μg/ml of CB. The increase of CD8+ cells in MLR was suppressed by addition of CB and cytotoxicity targeting the allo-PBMC using sorted CD8+ cells after cultivation was also reduced. Consistent with these findings, intracellular positivity of effector molecules such as granzyme B and interferon (IFN)-γ in CD8+ cells cultured with CB during the MLR was reduced. Regarding the differentiation of CD8+ cells, CD45RA as the marker for naïve CD8+ cells remained relatively high, while CD25 and CD45RO as markers of effector/memory CD8+ cells were not elevated when cultured with CB, compared with no CB MLR. In addition, the proliferation of CD8+ cells examined by the carboxyfluorescein succinimidyl ester (CFSE) labeling method was also inhibited when cultured with CB, although apoptotic cells of CD8+ cells were not changed regardless of whether the MLR was cocultured with or without CB. Furthermore, production of tumor necrosis factor (TNF)-α and IFN-γ in culture supernatants decreased when MLR was performed with CB, whereas IL-2 did not change irrespective of the presence of CB. These findings show that asbestos exposure causes inhibitory effects on CTL induction from CD8+ naïve T cells [29–31].

1.2.2.2   Characteristics of CTL in Asbestos-Exposed Patients

CTL differentiation and proliferation were impaired by asbestos exposure in asbestos-exposed patients with MM and pleural plaque (PP), who showed plaque in pleura as the marker of asbestos exposure and no other health effects in their body. The status of CTL characteristics in PP and MM patients was not identical. Analysis of CD8+ cells from PP patients revealed an increase of the perforin-positive and CD45RA-negative population in peripheral blood, as well as an increase of the per-forin- and IFN-γ-positive fraction after in vitro stimulation, whereas MM patients showed a decrease of perforin-positive CD8+ cells in peripheral blood. Furthermore, this reduction was not due to the excess degranulation.

Details regarding the features of CTL in PP and MM were published in our previous reports. In particular, the reduction of killing activity in CD8+ cells caused by asbestos exposure suggests that the pathophysiological status such as the presence or absence of cancers may alter the function of CTL. This issue needs to be resolved in future studies [29–31].

1.2.3   Alteration of T Cell Caused by Asbestos Exposure

1.2.3.1   T Helper 1 (Th1) Cell

Asbestos Exposure on Human T Cell Line, MT-2

A human T cell line, MT-2 (human T cell leukemia/lymphoma virus 1 (HTLV-1) immortalized polyclonal T cell line), was utilized to establish a continuous and recurrent asbestos exposure model (more than 1 year exposure to low-dose asbestos fibers and details were reported previously [32]). Six independent continuously exposed sublines of MT-2 cocultured with CB were established, and cDNA micro-array analysis was performed to compare the sublines with the original MT-2 cells, which were never exposed to asbestos. All six sublines showed a similar expression pattern of cDNA, and 84 up- and 55 downregulated genes were specified. Network analysis using the MetaCore™ system indicated that the IFN-γ pathway was involved in the sublines. All sublines showed a decrease in IFN regulatory factor 9 (IRF9) and IFN-stimulating gene factor 3 (ISGF3), as well as a decrease of CXC chemo-kine receptor 3 (CXCR3), which was regulated by IRF9. Since it is known that the Th1 cell shows higher IFN-γ and CXCR3 expression, mRNA and protein expression in the MT-2 sublines were reanalyzed. Results indicated that all sublines showed a decrease of CXCR3 and IFN-γ productive capacity, whereas the other Th1-type chemokine receptor, C-C chemokine receptor type 5 (CCR5) which had been chosen as the comparison, did not change [33–35].

CXCR3 and IFN-γ in Peripheral Th1 Cells Cultured with CB

Following analysis of the cell line model, in which it was supposed that asbestos exposure may inhibit Th1 function, and to confirm these findings in freshly isolated CD4+ Th cells from HD, these cells were stimulated and activated using anti-CD3 and anti-CD28 antibodies with IL-2 and cocultured with or without 5 or 10 μg/ml of CB. The CB-exposed Th cells showed decreased surface and mRNA expression of CXCR3 and intracellular IFN-γ-positive cells after 4 weeks of cultivation. These results indicated that ex vivo exposure to asbestos causes a distinct reduction of Th1 function as revealed by expression of CXCR3 and IFN-γ [33–35].

CXCR3 Expression of Peripheral CD4+ Cells in MM and PP Patients

In response to the experimental results of the cell culture, the expressions of CXCR3 and IFN-γ were analyzed in peripheral blood CD4+ cells derived from PP and MM patients, and results were compared with those from HD. Results showed that the CXCR3 expression level in CD4+ cells from PP and MM patients decreased and that of MM was lower than that of PP, whereas expression of CD4+CCR5+ cells in peripheral blood did not differ between the PP, MM, and HD groups. Moreover, CD4+ Th cells derived from MM showed decreased mRNA expression of IFN-γ when cells were ex vivo stimulated. A consideration of the overall results and experimental findings indicates that clinical exposure to asbestos induces dysfunction of Th1 cells as specifically revealed by decreased expression of CXCR3 and IFN-γ. Since both CXCR3 and IFN-γ are known to be important for antitumor immunity, these findings support the hypothesis that asbestos exposure induces a gradual decrease of antitumor immunity in the body of an exposed individual, which eventually causes lung cancer and MM in these individuals after a long latent period following the initial exposure to asbestos [33–35].

1.2.3.2   Regulatory T Cell (Treg)

In Vitro Assessment of Treg Function Exposed to Asbestos Using MT-2

The MT-2 cell line is known to possess Treg functionality, since HTLV-1 has a high affinity for Treg cells and adult T cell leukemia/lymphoma is considered a malignancy of Treg [36–38]. Treg is important for various pathophysiological states; for example, if the quality or quantity of Treg is decreased, allergy and autoimmune disorders may occur because the reaction of responder T cells against self- or non-self-antigens is not suppressed by Treg. In addition, if the function or volume of Treg is upregulated, antitumor immunity may decrease because responder T cells that recognize the tumor antigen and CTL suppress their function [39–41].

The abovementioned cell line model continuously exposed to asbestos was established using MT-2, and analyses of Treg function using the MT-2 sublines and the original MT-2 cell line, which was never exposed to asbestos fibers, may clarify the alteration of Treg following asbestos exposure [42].

Treg expresses suppressive activity by cell-cell contact and soluble factors, typically known as IL-10 and transforming growth factor (TGF)β. Interestingly, all sublines showed overproduction of IL-10 and TGFβ. The overproduced IL-10 was regulated by Src family kinases in MT-2 because of the reduction of IL-10 production and expression by the Src family inhibitor 4-amino-5-(4-chlorophenyl)-7-(t-butyl)pyrazolo[3,4-d]pyrimidine (PP2). This IL-10 was utilized by MT-2 cells through autocrine mechanisms and caused phosphorylated activation of signal transducer and activator of transcription (STAT)3, as well as Bcl-2 located downstream of STAT3. These conditions made the sublines resistant to asbestos-induced apoptosis. In addition, the overproduced TGFβ resulted in TGFβ-induced growth inhibition in MT-2 original cells, with over-phosphorylation of the downstream signaling molecule p38, as well as the TGF pathway signaling molecule SMAD3, but resulted in a decrease of SMAD2 [32, 43].

The contact inhibitory function of the MT-2 sublines exposed continuously to asbestos was then examined. Freshly isolated CD4+ cells were stimulated with anti-CD3 and auto-peripheral blood monocyte-derived dendritic cells to induce proliferation of cells. Instead of autologous Treg, irradiated cells from the original MT-2 cell line or an asbestos-exposed subline were added to this culture. Results revealed that the subline showed a greater enhanced suppressive activity than the original MT-2 cells, indicating that asbestos exposure caused an increase of Treg function [42].

Furthermore, the overproduced soluble factors IL-10 and TGFβ were evaluated by individually knocking down both cytokines using the siRNA method. The abovementioned assay for Treg suppressive function was then performed using a transwell culture plate with the MT-2 subline, MT-2 original cells, and IL-10 or TGFβ knocked-down sublines and permitting only the soluble factor to affect CD4+ cell proliferation activity. Results indicated that the IL-10 and TGFβ knocked-down sublines had reduced suppressive activity. These findings show that asbestos-exposed Treg exhibits an enhanced inhibitory function by a cell-cell contact mechanism, as well as excess production of functional soluble factors [42].

Analysis of the number and/or function of Treg may be better for an evaluation of tumor-surrounding Treg, although we have not had the opportunity to analyze Treg surrounding MM or asbestos-induced lung cancer cells. Our current findings are therefore limited due to the experimental assay. However, asbestos may cause the reduction of antitumor immunity by altering Treg function. The examination of the level of proliferating activity and inhibitory function of Treg should be performed in future investigations [42].

1.3   Summary of Asbestos-Induced Reduction of Antitumor Immunity

Table 1.1 summarizes investigation of the experimental immunological effects of asbestos exposure on various immune cells and alteration of immune function in asbestos-exposed patients with PP and MM. Additionally, Fig. 1.1 summarizes the typical findings described in this chapter.

As mentioned at the beginning of this chapter, the carcinogenic actions of asbestos fibers are attributed to (1) oxygen stress, (2) chromosome tangling, and (3) absorption of other carcinogens in the lung [16–20]. Due to these or other mechanisms, mesothelial cells may tend to change their cellular and molecular characteristics toward an abnormal and transformed cell type. For example, p16 cyclin-dependent kinase inhibitor, NF2, neurofibromatosis type 2, BAP1, and breast cancer susceptibility gene 1 (BRCA1)-associated protein-1 (ubiquitin carboxyterminal hydrolase) are the typical altered tumor suppressor genes in MM [44–48]. However, many of these transforming cells are usually monitored by immune surveillance and then removed from the body. However, asbestos-exposed individuals may possess an impaired immune surveillance system as described in this chapter,

Table 1.1 Investigations of the experimental immunological effects of asbestos exposure on immune cells and alteration of immune function in asbestos-exposed patients

Immune cell type	Kinds of asbestos fiber for exposure or analyzed patients exposed to asbestos	Findings	References
NK cell			[23–28]
Human NK cell line, YT-A1	Cultivation with chrysotile	Reduction of cytotoxicity	
		Reduction of surface expression of NKG2D and 2B4	
		Decreased phosphorylation of ERK signaling molecule	
Peripheral CD56+ NK cells	Malignant mesothelioma	Low cytotoxicity	
		Low surface expression of NKp46-activating receptor	
Freshly isolated NK cells derived from healthy donors	Cultivation with chrysotile during in vitro activation	Reduction of surface expression of NKp46	
Cytotoxic T cell			[29–31]
Human CD8+ cells in mixed lymphocyte reaction (MLR)	Cultivation with chrysotile during MLR	Reduction of allogenic cell killing	
		Decrease of intracellular IFN-γ and granzyme B	
Peripheral CD8+ T cell	Pleural plaque	Relatively high perforin+ cell	

(continued)

Table 1.1 (continued)

Immune cell type	Kinds of asbestos fiber for exposure or analyzed patients exposed to asbestos	Findings	References
T helper cell			[32–34, 42, 43]
Human T cell line, MT-2	Continuous cultivation with chrysotile	Acquisition of asbestos-induced apoptosis	
		Excess expression and production of IL-10	
		Overexpression of Bcl-2	
		Reduced production of IFN-γ, TNF-α, and CXCL10	
		Reduction of CXCR3 surface and mRNA expressions	
		Hyperphosphorylation of β-actin	
		Excess binding capacity to chrysotile in vimentin, myosin 9, and tubulinβ2	
		Excess production of TGFβ with phosphorylation of p38 and SMAD3	
		Resistance to TGFβ-induced growth inhibition	
	Continuous cultivation with crocidolite	Acquisition of asbestos-induced apoptosis	
		Excess expression and production of IL-10	
		Enhancement of Bcl-2/Bax expression ratio	
		Reduced production of IFN-γ and TNF-α	
Freshly isolated CD4+ cells derived from healthy donors	Cultivation with chrysotile during in vitro activation	Reduced expression of surface CXCR3	
		Reduction of intracellular IFN-γ	
Peripheral CD4+ T cell	Pleural plaque	Low expression of surface CXCR3	
	Malignant mesothelioma	Remarkably lower expression of surface CXCR3	
		Low IFN-γ mRNA expression	
		High Bcl-2 mRNA expression	
Regulatory T cell			[41]
Human T cell line, MT-2	Continuous cultivation with chrysotile	Enhanced suppressive activity in cell-cell contact assay	
		Enhanced production of functional soluble factors such as IL-10 and TGFβ	

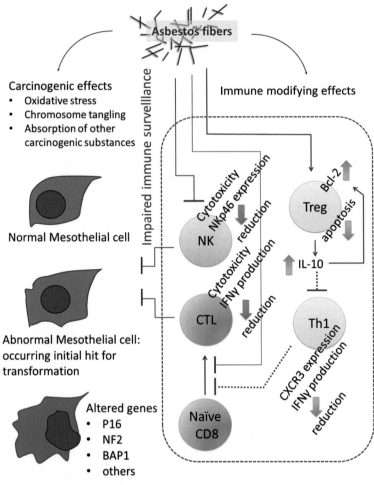

Fig. 1.1 Summarized schematic effects of asbestos fibers on various immune cells such as natural killer (NK), cytotoxic T lymphocyte (CTL), naïve CD8+, T helper 1 (Th1), and regulatory T (Treg) cells (*right side* of figure). The carcinogenic effects of asbestos fibers are shown on the *left side*, and normal mesothelial cells are gradually transformed toward malignant mesothelioma cells with alteration of tumor suppressor genes such as p16, NF2, and BAP1. Between these two effects, the usual immune surveillance system regarding cancerous cells may be impaired by asbestos exposure

and this impairment may result in MM and other cancers in these individuals after a long latent period [49–53].

Future investigations aimed at neutralizing the immune surveillance system in the asbestos-exposed population through physiologically active substances in foods, plants, and other materials are necessary in order to prevent the occurrence of cancerous diseases in asbestos-exposed individuals.

Acknowledgments The authors thank Ms. Minako Katoh, Naomi Miyahara, Satomi Hatada, Keiko Yamashita, Keiko Kimura, Tomoko Sueishi, and Misao Kuroki for their technical assistance. All the experimental findings performed in the Department of Hygiene, Kawasaki Medical School, were supported by the Special Coordination Fund for Promoting Science and Technology grant H18-1-3-3-1; JSPS KAKENHI grants 17790375, 19790431, 20890270, 22790550, 23790679, 24590770, and 25860470; Kawasaki Medical School Project grants 29-403, 19-407 M, 20-402O, 20411I, 32-107, 21-401, 22A29, 22B1, 23P3, 23B66, 24B39, and 25B41; the Kawasaki Foundation for Medical Science and Medical Welfare (2007 and 2009); and the Ryobi Teien Memorial Foundation (2009 and 2010).

References

1. Roggli VL, Coin P. Mineralogy of asbestos. In: Roggi VL, Oury TD, Sporn TA, editors. Pathology of asbestos-associated diseases. New York: Springer; 2004. p. 1–16.
2. Craighead JE, Gibbs A, Pooley F. Mineralogy of asbestos. In: Craighead JE, Gibbs AR, editors. Asbestos and its diseases. New York: Oxford University Press; 2008. p. 23–38.
3. Henderson DW, Leigh J. The history of asbestos utilization and recognition of asbestos-induced diseases. In: Dodson RF, Hammar SO, editors. Asbestos. Risk assessment, epidemiology, and health effects. 2nd ed. Boca Raton: CRC Press; 2011. p. 1–22.
4. Kohyama N, Shinohara Y, Suzuki Y. Mineral phases and some reexamined characteristics of the International Union Against Cancer standard asbestos samples. Am J Ind Med. 1996;30:515–28.
5. http://monographs.iarc.fr/ENG/Monographs/vol100C/mono100C.pdf
6. IARC monograph. A review of human carcinogens: arsenic, metals, fibres, and dusts (Iarc Monographs on the Evaluation of the Carcinogenic Risks to Humans). Geneva: World Health Organization; 2012.
7. Le GV, Takahashi K, Park EK, Delgermaa V, Oak C, Qureshi AM, Aljunid SM. Asbestos use and asbestos-related diseases in Asia: past, present and future. Respirology. 2011;16:767–75. doi:10.1111/j.1440-1843.2011.01975.x.
8. Kameda T, Takahashi K, Kim R, Jiang Y, Movahed M, Park EK, Rantanen J. Asbestos: use, bans and disease burden in Europe. Bull World Health Organ. 2014;92:790–7. doi:10.2471/BLT.13.132118.
9. O'Bryne K, Rusch V, editors. Malignant pleural mesothelioma. New York: Oxford University Press; 2006.
10. Hammar SP. Asbestos and mesothelioma. In: Dodson RF, Hammar SO, editors. Asbestos. Risk assessment, epidemiology, and health effects. 2nd ed. Boca Raton: CRC Press; 2011. p. 307–418.
11. Gibbs AR, Craighead JE. Malignant diseases of the pleura, peritoneum, and other serosal surface. In: Craighead JE, Gibbs AR, editors. Asbestos and its diseases. New York: Oxford University Press; 2008. p. 190–229.
12. Gibb H, Fulcher K, Nagarajan S, McCord S, Fallahian NA, Hoffman HJ, Haver C, Tolmachev S. Analyses of radiation and mesothelioma in the US transuranium and uranium registries. Am J Public Health. 2013;103:710–6. doi:10.2105/AJPH.2012.300928.
13. Emri R, Tuncer M, Baris YI. Malignant pleural mesothelioma in Turkey. In: O'Bryne K, Rusch V, editors. Malignant pleural mesothelioma. New York: Oxford University Press; 2006. p. 27–33.
14. Dikensoy O. Mesothelioma due to environmental exposure to erionite in Turkey. Curr Opin Pulm Med. 2008;14:322–5. doi:10.1097/MCP.0b013e3282fcea65.
15. Carbone M, Emri S, Dogan AU, Steele I, Tuncer M, Pass HI, Baris YI. A mesothelioma epidemic in Cappadocia: scientific developments and unexpected social outcomes. Nat Rev Cancer. 2007;7:147–54.

16. Pezerat H, Zalma R, Guignard J, Jaurand MC. Production of oxygen radicals by the reduction of oxygen arising from the surface activity of mineral fibres. IARC Sci Publ. 1989;90:100–11.

17. Neri M, Ugolini D, Dianzani I, Gemignani F, Landi S, Cesario A, Magnani C, Mutti L, Puntoni R, Bonassi S. Genetic susceptibility to malignant pleural mesothelioma and other asbestos-associated diseases. Mutat Res. 2008;659:126–36. doi:10.1016/j.mrrev.2008.02.002.

18. Liu G, Cheresh P, Kamp DW. Molecular basis of asbestos-induced lung disease. Annu Rev Pathol. 2013;8:161–87. doi:10.1146/annurev-pathol-020712-163942.

19. Toyokuni S. Mechanisms of asbestos-induced carcinogenesis. Nagoya J Med Sci. 2009;71:1–10.

20. Chew SH, Toyokuni S. Malignant mesothelioma as an oxidative stress-induced cancer: an update. Free Radic Biol Med. 2015;86:166–78. doi:10.1016/j.

21. Dodson RF, Williams Jr MG, Corn CJ, Brollo A, Bianchi C. A comparison of asbestos burden in lung parenchyma, lymph nodes, and plaques. Ann N Y Acad Sci. 1991;643:53–60.

22. Dodson RF, Huang J, Bruce JR. Asbestos content in the lymph nodes of nonoccupationally exposed individuals. Am J Ind Med. 2000;37:169–74.

23. Nishimura Y, Miura Y, Maeda M, Kumagai N, Murakami S, Hayashi H, Fukuoka K, Nakano T, Otsuki T. Impairment in cytotoxicity and expression of NK cell- activating receptors on human NK cells following exposure to asbestos fibers. Int J Immunopathol Pharmacol. 2009;22:579–90.

24. Nishimura Y, Maeda M, Kumagai N, Hayashi H, Miura Y, Otsuki T. Decrease in phosphorylation of ERK following decreased expression of NK cell-activating receptors in human NK cell line exposed to asbestos. Int J Immunopathol Pharmacol. 2009;22:879–88.

25. Nishimura Y, Kumagai N, Maeda M, Hayashi H, Fukuoka K, Nakano T, Miura Y, Hiratsuka J, Otsuki T. Suppressive effect of asbestos on cytotoxicity of human NK cells. Int J Immunopathol Pharmacol. 2011;24:5S–10.

26. Nishimura Y, Maeda M, Kumagai-Takei N, Lee S, Matsuzaki H, Wada Y, Nishiike-Wada T, Iguchi H, Otsuki T. Altered functions of alveolar macrophages and NK cells involved in asbestos-related diseases. Environ Health Prev Med. 2013;18:198–204. doi:10.1007/s12199-013-0333-y.

27. Nishimura Y, Kumagai-Takei N, Matsuzaki H, Lee S, Maeda M, Kishimoto T, Fukuoka K, Nakano T, Otsuki T. Functional alteration of natural killer cells and cytotoxic T lymphocytes upon asbestos exposure and in malignant mesothelioma patients. Biomed Res Int. 2015;2015:238431. doi:10.1155/2015/238431.

28. Nishimura Y, Maeda M, Kumagai-Takei N, Matsuzaki H, Lee S, Fukuoka K, Nakano T, Kishimoto T, Otsuki T. Effect of asbestos on anti-tumor immunity and immunological alteration in patients with mesothelioma. In: Belli C, Santosh Anand S, editors. Malignant mesothelioma. Rijeka: InTech Open Access Publisher; 2012. doi:10.5772/33138.

29. Kumagai-Takei N, Nishimura Y, Maeda M, Hayashi H, Matsuzaki H, Lee S, Hiratsuka J, Otsuki T. Effect of asbestos exposure on differentiation of cytotoxic T lymphocytes in mixed lymphocyte reaction of human peripheral blood mononuclear cells. Am J Respir Cell Mol Biol. 2013;49:28–36. doi:10.1165/rcmb.2012-0134OC.

30. Kumagai-Takei N, Nishimura Y, Maeda M, Hayashi H, Matsuzaki H, Lee S, Kishimoto T, Fukuoka K, Nakano T, Otsuki T. Functional properties of CD8(+) lymphocytes in patients with pleural plaque and malignant mesothelioma. J Immunol Res. 2014;2014:670140. doi:10.1155/2014/670140.

31. Kumagai-Takei N, Nishimura Y, Matsuzaki H, Maeda M, Lee S, Yoshitome K, Otsuki T. Effects of asbestos fibers on human cytotoxic T cells. In: Otsuki T, Holian A, Yoshioka Y, editors. Biological effects of fibrous and particulate substances, Current topics in environmental health and preventive medicine. Tokyo: Springer Japan; 2015. p. 211–21.

32. Miura Y, Nishimura Y, Katsuyama H, Maeda M, Hayashi H, Dong M, Hyodoh F, Tomita M, Matsuo Y, Uesaka A, Kuribayashi K, Nakano T, Kishimoto T, Otsuki T. Involvement of IL-10

and Bcl-2 in resistance against an asbestos-induced apoptosis of T cells. Apoptosis. 2006;11:1825–35.

33. Maeda M, Nishimura Y, Hayashi H, Kumagai N, Chen Y, Murakami S, Miura Y, Hiratsuka J, Kishimoto T, Otsuki T. Reduction of CXC chemokine receptor 3 in an *in vitro* model of continuous exposure to asbestos in a human T-cell line, MT-2. Am J Respir Cell Mol Biol. 2011;45:470–9. doi:10.1165/rcmb.2010-0213OC.

34. Maeda M, Nishimura Y, Hayashi H, Kumagai N, Chen Y, Murakami S, Miura Y, Hiratsuka J, Kishimoto T, Otsuki T. Decreased CXCR3 expression in CD4+ T cells exposed to asbestos or derived from asbestos-exposed patients. Am J Respir Cell Mol Biol. 2011;45:795–803. doi:10.1165/rcmb.2010-0435OC.

35. Maeda M, Yamamoto S, Hatayama T, Mastuzaki H, Lee S, Kumagai-Takei N, Yoshitome K, Nishimura Y, Kimura Y, Otsuki T. T cell alteration caused by exposure to asbestos. In: Otsuki T, Holian A, Yoshioka Y, editors. Biological effects of fibrous and particulate substances, Current topics in environmental health and preventive medicine. Tokyo: Springer Japan; 2015. p. 195–210.

36. Hamano R, Wu X, Wang Y, Oppenheim JJ, Chen X. Characterization of MT-2 cells as a human regulatory T cell-like cell line. Cell Mol Immunol. 2015;12:780–2. doi:10.1038/cmi.2014.123.

37. Chen S, Ishii N, Ine S, Ikeda S, Fujimura T, Ndhlovu LC, Soroosh P, Tada K, Harigae H, Kameoka J, Kasai N, Sasaki T, Sugamura K. Regulatory T cell-like activity of Foxp3+ adult T cell leukemia cells. Int Immunol. 2006;18:269–77.

38. Shimauchi T, Kabashima K, Tokura Y. Adult T-cell leukemia/lymphoma cells from blood and skin tumors express cytotoxic T lymphocyte-associated antigen-4 and Foxp3 but lack suppressor activity toward autologous CD8+ T cells. Cancer Sci. 2008;99:98–106.

39. Sakaguchi S. Naturally arising Foxp3-expressing CD25+CD4+ regulatory T cells in immunological tolerance to self and non-self. Nat Immunol. 2005;6:345–52.

40. Yamaguchi T, Sakaguchi S. Regulatory T cells in immune surveillance and treatment of cancer. Semin Cancer Biol. 2006;16:115–23.

41. Miyara M, Sakaguchi S. Natural regulatory T cells: mechanisms of suppression. Trends Mol Med. 2007;13:108–16.

42. Ying C, Maeda M, Nishimura Y, Kumagai-Takei N, Hayashi H, Matsuzaki H, Lee S, Yoshitome K, Yamamoto S, Hatayama T, Otsuki T. Enhancement of regulatory T cell-like suppressive function in MT-2 by long-term and low-dose exposure to asbestos. Toxicology. 2015;338:86–94. doi:10.1016/j.tox.2015.10.005.

43. Maeda M, Chen Y, Hayashi H, Kumagai-Takei N, Matsuzaki H, Lee S, Nishimura Y, Otsuki T. Chronic exposure to asbestos enhances TGF-β1 production in the human adult T cell leukemia virus-immortalized T cell line MT-2. Int J Oncol. 2014;45:2522–32. doi:10.3892/ijo.2014.2682.

44. Sekido Y. Genomic abnormalities and signal transduction dysregulation in malignant mesothelioma cells. Cancer Sci. 2010;101:1–6. doi:10.1111/j.1349-7006.2009.01336.x.

45. Sekido Y. Inactivation of Merlin in malignant mesothelioma cells and the Hippo signaling cascade dysregulation. Pathol Int. 2011;61:331–44. doi:10.1111/j.1440-1827.2011.02666.x.

46. Sekido Y. Molecular pathogenesis of malignant mesothelioma. Carcinogenesis. 2013;34(7):1413–9. doi:10.1093/carcin/bgt166.

47. Cheung M, Talarchek J, Schindeler K, Saraiva E, Penney LS, Ludman M, Testa JR. Further evidence for germline BAP1 mutations predisposing to melanoma and malignant mesothelioma. Cancer Genet. 2013;206:206–10. doi:10.1016/j.cancergen.2013.05.018.

48. Singhi AD, Krasinskas AM, Choudry HA, Bartlett DL, Pingpank JF, Zeh HJ, Luvison A, Fuhrer K, Bahary N, Seethala RR, Dacic S. The prognostic significance of BAP1, NF2, and CDKN2A in malignant peritoneal mesothelioma. Mod Pathol. 2016;29:14–24. doi:10.1038/modpathol.2015.121.

49. Otsuki T, Maeda M, Murakami S, Hayashi H, Miura Y, Kusaka M, Nakano T, Fukuoka K, Kishimoto T, Hyodoh F, Ueki A, Nishimura Y. Immunological effects of silica and asbestos. Cell Mol Immunol. 2007;4:261–8.

50. Maeda M, Nishimura Y, Kumagai N, Hayashi H, Hatayama T, Katoh M, Miyahara N, Yamamoto S, Hirastuka J, Otsuki T. Dysregulation of the immune system caused by silica and asbestos. J Immunotoxicol. 2010;7:268–78. doi:10.3109/1547691X.2010.512579.
51. Kumagai-Takei N, Maeda M, Chen Y, Matsuzaki H, Lee S, Nishimura Y, Hiratsuka J, Otsuki T. Asbestos induces reduction of tumor immunity. Clin Dev Immunol. 2011;2011:481439. doi:10.1155/2011/481439.
52. Matsuzaki H, Maeda M, Lee S, Nishimura Y, Kumagai-Takei N, Hayashi H, Yamamoto S, Hatayama T, Kojima Y, Tabata R, Kishimoto T, Hiratsuka J, Otsuki T. Asbestos-induced cellular and molecular alteration of immunocompetent cells and their relationship with chronic inflammation and carcinogenesis. J Biomed Biotechnol. 2012;2012:492608. doi:10.1155/2012/492608.
53. Otsuki T, Matsuzaki H, Lee S, Kumagai-Takei N, Yamamoto S, Hatayama T, Yoshitome K, Nishimura Y. Environmental factors and human health: fibrous and particulate substance-induced immunological disorders and construction of a health-promoting living environment. Environ Heallth Prev Med. 2015;21:71–81. doi:10.1007/s12199-015-0499-6.

Chapter 2
Silica-Induced Immunotoxicity: Chronic and Aberrant Activation of Immune Cells

Suni Lee, Hiroaki Hayashi, Hidenori Matsuzaki, Naoko Kumagai-Takei, Megumi Maeda, Kei Yoshitome, Shoko Yamamoto, Tamayo Hatayama, Yasumitsu Nishimura, and Takemi Otsuki

Abstract Occupational and chronic exposure to silica particles causes pulmonary fibrosis known as silicosis, which is a typical form of pneumoconiosis. Although the respiratory complications of silicosis include pulmonary tuberculosis, pleurisy, bronchitis, and other disorders such as lung cancer, silicosis (SIL) patients often suffer from complications of autoimmune diseases such as rheumatoid arthritis (RA), systemic sclerosis (SSc), and other forms of these conditions. The mechanisms causing impairment of immunity by silica exposure were considered adjuvant effects of these particles, and we have been investigating the direct effects of particles on immune cells, particularly T cells, and found chronic activation of both responder and regulatory T helper cells. The results of chronic activation indicated that responder T cells obtain resistance against CD95/Fas-mediated apoptosis to survive longer, whereas regulatory T cells become prone to CD95/Fas-mediated apoptosis and die quickly. These findings suggest that the imbalance of these cells may initiate the observed autoimmune disorders. Furthermore, various autoantibodies were detected in the serum of SIL without any symptoms of autoimmune diseases. Further investigation is needed to study the effects of silica on other immune cell types such as Th17, dendritic, and B cells. Adequate preventive tools against the progression of immunological impairments are also required to improve occupational health.

S. Lee • H. Matsuzaki • N. Kumagai-Takei • K. Yoshitome • S. Yamamoto • T. Hatayama
Y. Nishimura • T. Otsuki (✉)
Department of Hygiene, Kawasaki Medical School,
577 Matsushima, Kurashiki, Okayama 701-0192, Japan
e-mail: takemi@med.kawasaki-m.ac.jp

H. Hayashi
Department of Dermatology, Kawasaki Medical School,
577 Matsushima, Kurashiki, Okayama 701-0192, Japan

M. Maeda
Department of Biofunctional Chemistry, Division of Bioscience, Okayama University
Graduate School of Natural Science and Technology,
1-1-1 Tsushima-Naka, Kita-Ku, Okayama 7008530, Japan

© Springer Science+Business Media Singapore 2017
T. Otsuki et al. (eds.), *Allergy and Immunotoxicology in Occupational Health*,
Current Topics in Environmental Health and Preventive Medicine,
DOI 10.1007/978-981-10-0351-6_2

15

Keywords Silica • Autoimmune diseases • Regulatory T cell • CD95/Fas •
Apoptosis

2.1 Silica Exposure and Pulmonary Diseases

Silica-exposed patients suffer from pulmonary fibrosis known as silicosis, a typical
form of pneumoconiosis [1–5]. Although silicosis is divided clinically into chronic,
subacute, and acute forms, simple silicosis is characterized by the presence of small
rounded shadows, which usually appear in the upper lobes and later are observed
throughout the lungs [1–5]. This is a classic disease historically and was noted in the
era of Hippocrates, as well as Ramazzini and Agricola in their books *De Morbis
Artificum Diatriba* and *De Re Metallica* [1–3]. They wrote that miners developed
dyspnea and suggested a positive relationship between rock-dust exposure and dyspnea. The occupational sources of exposure are mining, quarrying (granite, sand-
stone, slate, pumice, pumicite), tunneling, stone working, activities involving
abrasives, glass manufacture, the agate industry and glass manufacture, the refractory brick industry, and many other sources [1–6].

The pulmonary complications of silicosis are typically tuberculosis, as well as
pleuritis, pneumothorax, bronchitis, bronchiectasis, and lung cancer. Interestingly,
the International Agency for Research on Cancer (IARC) of the World Health
Organization (WHO) categorized crystalline silica as a group I carcinogen when
inhaled in the form of quartz and cristobalite from occupational sources [7–10].

Basically, there are no curative procedures for chronic progression of lung fibrosis designated as silicosis, and these patients suffer from dyspnea and other pulmonary symptoms [1–5].

2.2 Immune Complications

In addition to the pulmonary complications mentioned above, SIL suffer from autoimmune disorders [1–3, 11–15]. Caplan's syndrome [16, 17] and rheumatoid arthritis (RA) are well-known complications of silicosis. Systemic sclerosis (SSc) [18–21]
and systemic lupus erythematosus (SLE) [22–24] are also known as frequent complications of silicosis, although SLE appears to be limited to workers associated
with sandblasting, grinding, and the handling of silica for use as a scouring powder
or in patients with acute or accelerated silicosis [1–3]. More recently, anti-neutrophil
cytoplasmic antibody (ANCA)-related vasculitis/nephritis have been reported as
complications in SIL [25–28].

Basically, the cellular mechanisms responsible for the dysregulation of autoimmunity caused by silica exposure have been regarded as an adjuvant effect of the
silica particles [29–31]. There are many self-antigens such as proteins, amino acids,

and nucleotides derived from cell debris yielded by physiological cell apoptosis and other processes in the body. These candidate antigens may bind with the silica particles as adjuvants and subsequently exert strong antigenicity to induce the autoimmune diseases observed in SIL.

However, since inhaled silica particles remain in the lung and lymph nodes, these particles may recurrently and chronically encounter circulating immune cells [1–5]. It is therefore reasonable to consider the possible direct effects of these inhaled silica particles on the peripheral immune cells of the human body.

2.3 Alteration of Immune Cells and Functions

2.3.1 Responder T Cell Activation Caused by Silica

Although it is commonly thought that immunotoxicity may kill immune-competent cells through the action of certain substances, our investigations have revealed excess immune stimulation or reduction of certain immune levels due to environmental factors such as silica particles to result in representative phenotypes of immunotoxicity when considering that immune systems should remain physiologically neutral. Excess immune reactions cause allergies and autoimmune disorders, and a reduced immunological state may result in impairment of tumor immunity and transplantation immunity. Thus, a consideration of immune impairments caused by environmental substances suggests that altered activation and/or reduced function of immune cells should be regarded as an indication of immunotoxicity in the broad sense of the term.

In vitro experiments were performed initially to determine whether silica particles produced immunotoxic effects on human peripheral T cells [32]. When peripheral blood mononuclear cells (PBMCs) were cultured with or without silica particles, only T cells in PBMC gradually expressed CD69 as an early activation marker of T cells for 4–10 days, although the increased expression of CD69 was slower than that of standard mitogen such as phytohemagglutinin (PHA), which immediately activated T cells within 24 h followed by cessation within 2 or 3 days. Actually, chrysotile asbestos fibers did not allow T cells to express CD69 [32].

In addition, PD-1 expression as one of the chronically activated T cell markers was examined using peripheral blood T cells (CD4+ and CD25+ or CD4+ CD25- fractions) from SIL and compared with that of healthy volunteers (HV). Both fractions derived from SIL showed a significantly higher expression of PD-1 than that of HV [33].

Since the concentration of serum soluble interleukin (IL)-2 receptor (sIL-2R) has recently been considered an activation marker of T cells in autoimmune diseases, in addition to tumor biomarker for T cell leukemia and lymphoma [34, 35], serum sIL-2R levels in HV, SIL, and SSc were measured and compared [36]. Results revealed that sIL-2R levels in SSc were significantly higher than those in HV, and levels in

SIL tended to be higher than those in HV. In addition, the level of sIL-2R in SIL was correlated with antinuclear antibody (ANA) titer, immunoglobulin (Ig) G, and anti-centromere/CENP-B antibody titer. Furthermore, factor analysis indicated that sIL-2R in SIL contributed to the subpopulation with a poorer immunological status without much impairment of respiratory parameters [36]. Thus, sIL-2R was also considered an indicator of the chronically activated status of T cells in SIL.

The overall findings suggested that responder T cells in SIL are chronically activated by recurrent encounters with silica particles in the circulation.

2.3.2 Inhibitory Molecules for CD95/Fas-Mediated Apoptosis in SIL

As mentioned above, responder T cells circulating in the peripheral blood of SIL are activated chronically. However, the reactions of activated T cells usually cease due to activation-induced cell death (AICD) mediated by CD95/Fas death receptor via autocrine or paracrine binding with Fas ligand produced by similarly activated T cells [37–39]. Examination of autoimmune diseases revealed that HV had lower serum levels of soluble Fas (sFas), which lacks the transmembrane domain of the Fas molecule as an alternatively spliced variant and is secreted from cells for binding with the auto- or para-produced Fas ligand at extracellular spaces to prevent Fas-mediated apoptosis/AICD [40–43]. If the chronically activated T cells in these diseases, which are recognizing the self-antigens, are avoiding AICD/Fas-mediated apoptosis, these self-recognizing T cells may survive longer and cause continuous impairment of autoimmunity to result in autoimmune disorders that last longer and progress to worsening states.

Serum sFas levels in SIL were also elevated, and examination of mRNA expression in PBMC revealed excess expression of the sFas message, which lacks the 63 bp of the transmembrane domain relative to the wild-type membrane and binds the Fas molecule [44, 45]. In addition, PBMC from SIL showed a higher expression relative to HV of other alternatively spliced variants of the Fas gene, all of which conserved the Fas-ligand binding domain but lacked the transmembrane domain [46]. Most of these variants may act in a manner similar to the typical variant, the sFas molecule, to prevent Fas-mediated apoptosis.

Similar to sFas, decoy receptor 3 (DcR3) was also found to prevent TNF-related apoptosis-inducing ligand (Trail)-mediated apoptosis by binding with Trail at extracellular spaces [47–49]. DcR3 molecules were first reported to be produced by lung and colon cancer cells for self-prevention from tumor attacking Trail secreted by T cells bearing tumor immunity [50]. Thereafter, serum DcR3 levels were found to be higher in various autoimmune diseases. In our analysis, PBMC from SIL showed a higher DcR3 expression level than that of HV [51]. We have been trying recently to measure serum DcR3 levels, as well as determine the role of DcR3 levels in the immunological pathophysiological status of SIL. We will report the findings of these investigations in the near future.

The overall results indicate that responder T cells chronically activated by silica particles avoid AICD/Fas-mediated apoptosis by self-producing inhibitory molecules.

2.3.3   Regulatory T Cells in Silicosis Peripheral Blood

When we consider the T cell status that tends to progress to autoimmune disorders, the balance between responder T cells and regulatory T cells (Treg) defined by CD4+ CD25+ and forkhead box P3 (FoxP3) transcription factor positive is important, and reduction of function and/or number of Treg may prolong the activation of responder T cells from various non-self or self-antigens and cause autoimmune disorders [52, 53]. In addition, T helper 17 (Th17) cells are also important in the formation of autoimmune disorders [54–56]. Cytokine levels, particularly those of IL-6 and transforming growth factor (TGF-)-β, influence the polarization between Treg and Th17 cells [57–59]. Although we have not investigated Th17 alteration following exposure to silica particles, we found an interesting change in Treg following exposure to silica particles, as well as alteration of peripheral Treg from SIL [60].

We first examined Treg function derived from the CD4+CD25+ fraction of SIL and compared it with that of HV [60]. Although the examined SIL did not show any symptoms of autoimmune diseases, the suppressive function that reduces the antigen-induced proliferation in responder (CD4+CD25-) T cells induced by a cocultured peripheral blood CD4+CD25+ fraction was reduced in SIL compared to HV. This result indicated that Treg function in the peripheral CD4+CD25+ fraction of SIL may be reduced or weakened by chronic exposure to silica particles [60].

Treg from SIL and HV showed higher CD95/Fas expression compared with that in responder T cells of the CD4+CD25- fraction [33]. However, it was significantly higher in SIL compared to HV. Since CD95/Fas expression in Treg is known as an activation marker for this cell type, chronic silica exposure may stimulate Treg in a manner similar to that of responder T cells as mentioned above. The results showing chronic activation of Treg with excess expression of CD95/Fas may indicate they are sensitive to Fas-mediated apoptosis [33]. In fact, Treg from SIL proceeded toward apoptosis more rapidly and with greater amounts compared to Treg from HV when these cells were cultured with agonistic anti-Fas antibody. Furthermore, cultures with silica particles and PBMCs from HV revealed that the CD4+CD25+ fraction as a marker of Treg and activated responder T cells did not change remarkably; however, the level of FoxP3+ in CD4+ decreased significantly during the culture period [33]. These results indicate that Treg in SIL are highly sensitive to Fas-mediated apoptosis and can be killed easily and may be recruited from the bone marrow [33].

The overall findings show that silica exposure chronically activates responder T cells and Treg. The former are resistant to Fas-mediated apoptosis and survive longer, whereas the latter are sensitive and progress toward cell death. An imbalance between these two types of T cells then occurs in SIL and subsequently results in the germination of impaired autoimmunity.

2.3.4   Autoantibodies in SIL

We have reported various autoantibodies that were found in SIL. For example, anti-CD95/Fas autoantibody was found in approximately one fourth of SIL [61]. This autoantibody was functional, i.e., when this autoantibody binds with membrane Fas, the cells proceed toward apoptosis. This was confirmed using sister human myeloma cell lines from pleural effusion and the bone marrow derived from the same patients [61, 62]. The cell line from the effusion showed scant Fas expression, whereas the line from the bone marrow exhibited strong expression. Additionally, the former line was not killed by serum from anti-Fas autoantibody positive SIL, but cells in the latter line died. These results indicated that Treg in SIL who are positive for this autoantibody are much more sensitive and likely to be killed.

We have also reported anti-caspase 8 [63, 64] and anti-desmoglein autoantibodies [65] in SIL. Moreover, anti-Scl-70 (topoisomerase I) autoantibody was detected in SIL [66, 67]. These autoantibodies are clinically significant and are often detected in SSc. The anti-Scl-70 autoantibody is seen in the diffuse SSc type with organ fibrosis such as the lung, whereas the anti-CENP-B (centromere) autoantibody is observed in the limited type of SSc with lesions in the esophagus and involving pulmonary hypertension. The clinical status of both antibodies was assayed in SIL patients that did not exhibit any symptoms of SSc. Recently, the titer index (Log_{10}) of anti-CENP-B autoantibody in SIL was higher than that of HV, and that of SSc was higher than those of HV and SIL. This titer index was positively correlated with an assumed immune status of one for HV, two for SIL, and three for SSc. Moreover, factor analysis of SIL cases revealed that although the titer index of anti-CENP-B autoantibody formed the same factor with that of anti-Scl-70 autoantibody, the Ig G value and the age of patients and other factors extracted showed that the Ig A value and anti-Scl-70 antibody were positively related, but anti-CENP-B showed an opposite tendency [68]. These results indicated that the titer index of anti-CENP-B autoantibody may be a biomarker for dysregulation in SIL cases.

Our findings suggest that B cells, as the producer of autoantibodies, may be affected by chronic silica exposure and an alteration caused by long-surviving responder T cells. In addition, dendritic cells as the initial antigen-presenting cell may have their function modified by chronic exposure to silica, although we have not performed a detailed analysis of the cellular and molecular alterations of these cells following silica exposure.

2.4 Conclusion

All the findings described above are summarized schematically in Fig. 2.1. Silica exposure causes a form of pulmonary fibrosis known as silicosis, a condition that progresses gradually to reduce the health of affected individuals. In addition, the pulmonary complications observed with this condition sometimes result in a severe pathological status, particularly when involving tuberculosis and lung cancer, which further burdens SIL patients with a difficult clinical course. However, silica

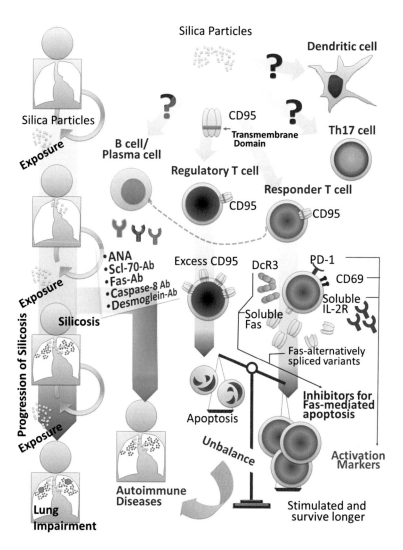

Fig. 2.1 Schematic presentation of the immunological effects of silica particles, particularly on responder T cells and regulatory T cells, and the detection of various autoantibodies

particles not only cause respiratory impairments, but also immunological disorders, especially those involving autoimmune diseases [68–74]. Based on the adjuvant effect of silica particles, our investigations have elucidated the direct action of silica on immune-competent cells. Silica chronically activates responder and regulatory T cells to result in an imbalance of these two types of T cells, which makes individuals more prone to developing autoimmune disorders. Once autoimmune impairments appear, the pathological status also progresses and worsens gradually, never to return to the previous unimpaired condition. Although future studies are required regarding silica's direct effects on Th17, dendritic, and B cells, investigations of preventive procedures using physiologically active substances or chemicals from plants and foods are necessary to inhibit the subclinical progression of immunological impairments and improve occupational health.

Acknowledgments The authors thank former colleagues in the Department of Hygiene, Kawasaki Medical School, namely, Prof. Ayako Ueki, Drs. Fuminori Hyodoh, Akiko Takata-Tomokuni, Yasuhiko Kawakami, Takaaki Aikoh, Shuko Murakami, and Yoshie Miura. We also appreciate the technical assistance of Ms. Haruko Sakaguchi, Naomi Miyahara, Minako Katoh, and Yumika Isozaki. We express special thanks to Drs. Masayasu Kusaka and Kozo Urakami for coordinating the collection of clinical samples. Part of the experimental results in this article was supported by the Special Coordination Fund for Promoting Science and Technology (H18-1-3-3-1, "Comprehensive approach on asbestos-related diseases"), KAKENHI grants (18390186, 19659153, 20390178, and 25460825), Kawasaki Medical School Project grants (20-410I, 23S5, 24S6, 25B65, and 27B06), the Sumitomo Foundation Grant (053027), the Yasuda Memorial Foundation Grant (H18), funding from the Takeda Science Foundation (I-2008) and Young Investigator Activating Grant from the Japanese Society of Hygiene (H18), the Ryobi Teien Memorial Foundation (H24), and the Kawasaki Foundation for Medical Science and Medical Welfare (H24).

References

1. Weill H, Jones RN, Raymond Parkes W. Silicosis and related diseases. In: Raymond Parkes W, editor. Occupational lung disorders. 3rd ed. Oxford: Butterworth-Heinemann Ltd; 1994. p. 285–339.
2. Weissman DN, Banks DE. Silicosis. In: Schwarz MI, King Jr TE, editors. Interstitial lung disease. 4th ed. Hamilton: BC Decker; 2003. p. 387–401.
3. Kelley J. Occupational lung diseases caused by asbestos, silica, and other silicates. In: Baum GL, Crapo JD, Celli BR, Karlinsky JB, editors. Textbook of pulmonary diseases, vol. 1. 6th ed. Philadelphia: Lippincott-Raven Publishers; 1998. p. 659–82.
4. Cullinan P, Reid P. Pneumoconiosis. Prim Care Respir J. 2013;22(2):249–52. doi:10.4104/pcrj.2013.00055.
5. Leung CC, Yu IT, Chen W. Silicosis. Lancet. 2012;379(9830):2008–18. doi:10.1016/S0140-6736(12)60235-9.
6. Rees D, Murray J. Silica, silicosis and tuberculosis. Int J Tuberc Lung Dis. 2007;11(5):474–84.
7. Silica, some silicates, coal dust and para-aramid fibrils. In: IARC monographs on the evaluation of carcinogenic risks to humans. Volume 68. Lyon: WHO Press. 1997.
8. Steenland K, Ward E. Silica: a lung carcinogen. CA Cancer J Clin. 2014;64(1):63–9. doi:10.3322/caac.21214.

9. Pelucchi C, Pira E, Piolatto G, Coggiola M, Carta P, La Vecchia C. Occupational silica exposure and lung cancer risk: a review of epidemiological studies 1996–2005. Ann Oncol. 2006;17(7):1039–50.

10. Finkelstein MM. Silica, silicosis, and lung cancer: a risk assessment. Am J Ind Med. 2000;38(1):8–18.

11. Uber CL, McReynolds RA. Immunotoxicology of silica. Crit Rev Toxicol. 1982;10(4):303–19.

12. Steenland K, Goldsmith DF. Silica exposure and autoimmune diseases. Am J Ind Med. 1995;28(5):603–8.

13. Mayes MD. Epidemiologic studies of environmental agents and systemic autoimmune diseases. Environ Health Perspect. 1999;107 Suppl 5:743–8.

14. Parks CG, Conrad K, Cooper GS. Occupational exposure to crystalline silica and autoimmune disease. Environ Health Perspect. 1999;107 Suppl 5:793–802.

15. Hess EV. Environmental chemicals and autoimmune disease: cause and effect. Toxicology. 2002;181–182:65–70.

16. Caplan A. Certain unusual radiological appearances in the chest of coal-miners suffering from rheumatoid arthritis. Thorax 8(1): 29–37. doi:10.1136/thx.8.1.29.

17. Caplan A. Rheumatoid disease and pneumoconiosis (Caplan's syndrome). Proc R Soc Med. 1959;52:1111–3.

18. Siltzbach LE. Diffuse pulmonary granulomatosis and fibroses. Mod Treat. 1964;15:290–306.

19. Rodnan GP, Benedek TG, Medsger Jr TA, Cammarata RJ. The association of progressive systemic sclerosis (scleroderma) with coal miners' pneumoconiosis and other forms of silicosis. Ann Intern Med. 1967;66(2):323–34.

20. Haustein UF, Ziegler V, Herrmann K, Mehlhorn J, Schmidt C. Silica-induced scleroderma. J Am Acad Dermatol. 1990;22(3):444–8.

21. Haustein UF, Anderegg U. Silica induced scleroderma – clinical and experimental aspects. J Rheumatol. 1998;25(10):1917–26.

22. Sanchez-Roman J, Wichmann I, Salaberri J, Varela JM, Nuñez-Roldan A. Multiple clinical and biological autoimmune manifestations in 50 workers after occupational exposure to silica. Ann Rheum Dis. 1993;52(7):534–8.

23. Koeger AC, Lang T, Alcaix D, Milleron B, Rozenberg S, Chaibi P, Arnaud J, Mayaud C, Camus JP, Bourgeois P. Silica-associated connective tissue disease. A study of 24 cases. Medicine (Baltimore). 1995;74(5):221–37.

24. D'Cruz D. Autoimmune diseases associated with drugs, chemicals and environmental factors. Toxicol Lett. 2000;112–113:421–32.

25. Gregorini G, Tira P, Frizza J, D'Haese PC, Elseviers MM, Nuyts G, Maiorca R, De Broe ME. ANCA-associated diseases and silica exposure. Clin Rev Allergy Immunol. 1997;15(1):21–40.

26. Tervaert JW, Stegeman CA, Kallenberg CG. Silicon exposure and vasculitis. Curr Opin Rheumatol. 1998;10(1):12–7.

27. Mulloy KB. Silica exposure and systemic vasculitis. Environ Health Perspect. 2003;111(16):1933–8.

28. Bartůnková J, Pelclová D, Fenclová Z, Sedivá A, Lebedová J, Tesar V, Hladíková M, Klusácková P. Exposure to silica and risk of ANCA-associated vasculitis. Am J Ind Med. 2006;49(7):569–76.

29. Levine S, Sowinski R. Enhancement of allergic encephalomyelitis by particulate adjuvants inoculated long before antigen. Am J Pathol. 1980;99(2):291–304.

30. Stone OJ. Autoimmunity as a secondary phenomenon in scleroderma (and so-called human adjuvant disease). Med Hypotheses. 1991;34(2):127–30.

31. Rao TD, Frey AB. Administration of silica sensitizes lipopolysaccharide responsiveness of murine macrophages but inhibits T and B cell priming by inhibition of antigen presenting function. Immunol Investig. 1998;27(3):181–99.

32. Wu P, Hyodoh F, Hatayama T, Sakaguchi H, Hatada S, Miura Y, Takata-Tomokuni A, Katsuyama H, Otsuki T. Induction of CD69 antigen expression in peripheral blood mononuclear cells on exposure to silica, but not by asbestos/chrysotile-A. Immunol Lett. 2005;98(1):145–52.
33. Hayashi H, Miura Y, Maeda M, Murakami S, Kumagai N, Nishimura Y, Kusaka M, Urakami K, Fujimoto W, Otsuki T. Reductive alteration of the regulatory function of the CD4(+) CD25(+) T cell fraction in silicosis patients. Int J Immunopathol Pharmacol. 2010;23(4):1099–109.
34. Witkowska AM. On the role of sIL-2R measurements in rheumatoid arthritis and cancers. Mediat Inflamm. 2005;2005(3):121–30.
35. Murakami S. Soluble interleukin-2 receptor in cancer. Front Biosci. 2004;9:3085–90.
36. Hayashi H, Maeda M, Murakami S, Kumagai N, Chen Y, Hatayama T, Katoh M, Miyahara N, Yamamoto S, Yoshida Y, Nishimura Y, Kusaka M, Fujimoto W, Otsuki T. Soluble interleukin-2 receptor as an indicator of immunological disturbance found in silicosis patients. Int J Immunopathol Pharmacol. 2009;22(1):53–62.
37. Kabelitz D, Janssen O. Antigen-induced death of T-lymphocytes. Front Biosci. 1997;2:d61–77.
38. Maher S, Toomey D, Condron C, Bouchier-Hayes D. Activation-induced cell death: the controversial role of Fas and Fas ligand in immune privilege and tumour counterattack. Immunol Cell Biol. 2002;80(2):131–7.
39. Green DR, Droin N, Pinkoski M. Activation-induced cell death in T cells. Immunol Rev. 2003;193:70–81.
40. Cheng J, Zhou T, Liu C, Shapiro JP, Brauer MJ, Kiefer MC, Barr PJ, Mountz JD. Protection from Fas-mediated apoptosis by a soluble form of the Fas molecule. Science. 1994;263(5154):1759–62.
41. Tokano Y, Miyake S, Kayagaki N, Nozawa K, Morimoto S, Azuma M, Yagita H, Takasaki Y, Okumura K, Hashimoto H. Soluble Fas molecule in the serum of patients with systemic lupus erythematosus. J Clin Immunol. 1996;16(5):261–5.
42. Jodo S, Kobayashi S, Kayagaki N, Ogura N, Feng Y, Amasaki Y, Fujisaku A, Azuma M, Yagita H, Okumura K, Koike T. Serum levels of soluble Fas/APO-1 (CD95) and its molecular structure in patients with systemic lupus erythematosus (SLE) and other autoimmune diseases. Clin Exp Immunol. 1997;107(1):89–95.
43. Nozawa K, Kayagaki N, Tokano Y, Yagita H, Okumura K, Hasimoto H. Soluble Fas (APO-1, CD95) and soluble Fas ligand in rheumatic diseases. Arthritis Rheum. 1997;40(6):1126–9.
44. Tomokuni A, Aikoh T, Matsuki T, Isozaki Y, Otsuki T, Kita S, Ueki H, Kusaka M, Kishimoto T, Ueki A. Elevated soluble Fas/APO-1 (CD95) levels in silicosis patients without clinical symptoms of autoimmune diseases or malignant tumours. Clin Exp Immunol. 1997;110(2):303–9.
45. Otsuki T, Sakaguchi H, Tomokuni A, Aikoh T, Matsuki T, Kawakami Y, Kusaka M, Ueki H, Kita S, Ueki A. Soluble Fas mRNA is dominantly expressed in cases with silicosis. Immunology. 1998;94(2):258–62.
46. Otsuki T, Sakaguchi H, Tomokuni A, Aikoh T, Matsuki T, Isozaki Y, Hyodoh F, Kawakami Y, Kusaka M, Kita S, Ueki A. Detection of alternatively spliced variant messages of Fas gene and mutational screening of Fas and Fas ligand coding regions in peripheral blood mononuclear cells derived from silicosis patients. Immunol Lett. 2000;72(2):137–43.
47. Yu KY, Kwon B, Ni J, Zhai Y, Ebner R, Kwon BS. A newly identified member of tumor necrosis factor receptor superfamily (TR6) suppresses LIGHT-mediated apoptosis. J Biol Chem. 1999;274(20):13733–6.
48. Lin WW, Hsieh SL. Decoy receptor 3: a pleiotropic immunomodulator and biomarker for inflammatory diseases, autoimmune diseases and cancer. Biochem Pharmacol. 2011;81(7):838–47. doi:10.1016/j.bcp.2011.01.011.

49. Siakavellas SI, Sfikakis PP, Bamias G. The TL1A/DR3/DcR3 pathway in autoimmune rheumatic diseases. Semin Arthritis Rheum. 2015;45(1):1–8. doi:10.1016/j.semarthrit.2015.02.007.
50. Pitti RM, Marsters SA, Lawrence DA, Roy M, Kischkel FC, Dowd P, Huang A, Donahue CJ, Sherwood SW, Baldwin DT, Godowski PJ, Wood WI, Gurney AL, Hillan KJ, Cohen RL, Goddard AD, Botstein D, Ashkenazi A. Genomic amplification of a decoy receptor for Fas ligand in lung and colon cancer. Nature. 1998;396(6712):699–703.
51. Otsuki T, Tomokuni A, Sakaguchi H, Aikoh T, Matsuki T, Isozaki Y, Hyodoh F, Ueki H, Kusaka M, Kita S, Ueki A. Over-expression of the decoy receptor 3 (DcR3) gene in peripheral blood mononuclear cells (PBMC) derived from silicosis patients. Clin Exp Immunol. 2000;119(2):323–7.
52. Sakaguchi S, Sakaguchi N, Shimizu J, Yamazaki S, Sakihama T, Itoh M, Kuniyasu Y, Nomura T, Toda M, Takahashi T. Immunologic tolerance maintained by CD25+ CD4+ regulatory T cells: their common role in controlling autoimmunity, tumor immunity, and transplantation tolerance. Immunol Rev. 2001;182:18–32.
53. Takahashi T, Sakaguchi S. Naturally arising CD25+CD4+ regulatory T cells in maintaining immunologic self-tolerance and preventing autoimmune disease. Curr Mol Med. 2003;3(8):693–706.
54. Afzali B, Lombardi G, Lechler RI, Lord GM. The role of T helper 17 (Th17) and regulatory T cells (Treg) in human organ transplantation and autoimmune disease. Clin Exp Immunol. 2007;148(1):32–46.
55. Chen Z, O'Shea JJ. Th17 cells: a new fate for differentiating helper T cells. Immunol Res. 2008;41(2):87–102. doi:10.1007/s12026-007-8014-9.
56. Korn T, Bettelli E, Oukka M, Kuchroo VK. IL-17 and Th17 Cells. Annu Rev Immunol. 2009;27:485–517. doi:10.1146/annurev.immunol.021908.132710.
57. O'Connor RA, Taams LS, Anderton SM. Translational mini-review series on Th17 cells: CD4 T helper cells: functional plasticity and differential sensitivity to regulatory T cell-mediated regulation. Clin Exp Immunol. 2010;159(2):137–47. doi:10.1111/j.1365-2249.2009.04040.x.
58. Girtsman T, Jaffar Z, Ferrini M, Shaw P, Roberts K. Natural Foxp3(+) regulatory T cells inhibit Th2 polarization but are biased toward suppression of Th17-driven lung inflammation. J Leukoc Biol. 2010;88(3):537–46. doi:10.1189/jlb.0110044.
59. Muranski P, Restifo NP. Essentials of Th17 cell commitment and plasticity. Blood. 2013;121(13):2402–14. doi:10.1182/blood-2012-09-378653.
60. Wu P, Miura Y, Hyodoh F, Nishimura Y, Hatayama T, Hatada S, Sakaguchi H, Kusaka M, Katsuyama H, Tomita M, Otsuki T. Reduced function of CD4+25+ regulatory T cell fraction in silicosis patients. Int J Immunopathol Pharmacol. 2006;19(2):357–68.
61. Takata-Tomokuni A, Ueki A, Shiwa M, Isozaki Y, Hatayama T, Katsuyama H, Hyodoh F, Fujimoto W, Ueki H, Kusaka M, Arikuni H, Otsuki T. Detection, epitope-mapping and function of anti-Fas autoantibody in patients with silicosis. Immunology. 2005;116(1):21–9.
62. Ohtsuki T, Yawata Y, Wada H, Sugihara T, Mori M, Namba M. Two human myeloma cell lines, amylase-producing KMS-12-PE and amylase-non-producing KMS-12-BM, were established from a patient, having the same chromosome marker, t(11;14)(q13;q32). Br J Haematol. 1989;73(2):199–204.
63. Ueki A, Isozaki Y, Tomokuni A, Hatayama T, Ueki H, Kusaka M, Shiwa M, Arikuni H, Takeshita T, Morimoto K. Intramolecular epitope spreading among anti-caspase-8 autoantibodies in patients with silicosis, systemic sclerosis and systemic lupus erythematosus, as well as in healthy individuals. Clin Exp Immunol. 2002;129(3):556–61.
64. Ueki A, Isozaki Y, Kusaka M. Anti-caspase-8 autoantibody response in silicosis patients is associated with HLA-DRB1, DQB1 and DPB1 alleles. J Occup Health. 2005;47(1):61–7.
65. Ueki H, Kohda M, Nobutoh T, Yamaguchi M, Omori K, Miyashita Y, Hashimoto T, Komai A, Tomokuni A, Ueki A. Antidesmoglein autoantibodies in silicosis patients with no bullous diseases. Dermatology. 2001;202(1):16–21.

66. Ueki A, Isozaki Y, Tomokuni A, Tanaka S, Otsuki T, Kishimoto T, Kusaka M, Aikoh T, Sakaguchi H, Hydoh F. Autoantibodies detectable in the sera of silicosis patients. The relationship between the anti-topoisomerase I antibody response and HLA-DQB1*0402 allele in Japanese silicosis patients. Sci Total Environ. 2001;270(1–3):141–8.

67. Tomokuni A, Otsuki T, Sakaguchi H, Isozaki Y, Hyodoh F, Kusaka M, Ueki A. Detection of anti-topoisomerase I autoantibody in patients with silicosis. Environ Health Prev Med. 2002;7(1):7–10. doi:10.1007/BF02898059.

68. Maeda M, Nishimura Y, Kumagai N, Hayashi H, Hatayama T, Katoh M, Miyahara N, Yamamoto S, Hirastuka J, Otsuki T. Dysregulation of the immune system caused by silica and asbestos. J Immunotoxicol. 2010;7(4):268–78. doi:10.3109/1547691X.2010.512579.

69. Lee S, Hayashi H, Maeda M, Chen Y, Matsuzaki H, Takei-Kumagai N, Nishimura Y, Fujimoto W, Otsuki T. Environmental factors producing autoimmune dysregulation – chronic activation of T cells caused by silica exposure. Immunobiology. 2012;217(7):743–8. doi:10.1016/j. imbio.2011.12.009.

70. Lee S, Matsuzaki H, Kumagai-Takei N, Yoshitome K, Maeda M, Chen Y, Kusaka M, Urakami K, Hayashi H, Fujimoto W, Nishimura Y, Otsuki T. Silica exposure and altered regulation of autoimmunity. Environ Health Prev Med. 2014;19(5):322–9. doi:10.1007/ s12199-014-0403-9.

71. Kumagai N, Hayashi H, Maeda M, Miura Y, Nishimura Y, Matsuzaki H, Lee S, Fujimoto W, Otsuki T. Immunological effects of silica and related dysregulation of autoimmunity. In: Mavragani CP, editor. Autoimmune disorders – pathogenetic aspects. Rijeka: InTech Open Access Publisher; 2011. p. 157–74.

72. Hayashi H, Nishimura Y, Hyodo F, Maeda M, Kumagai N, Miura Y, Kusaka M, Uragami K, Otsuki T. Dysregulation of autoimmunity caused by silica exposure: fas-mediated apoptosis in T lymphocytes derived from silicosis patients. In: Petri M, editor. Autoimmune disorders: symptoms, diagnosis and treatment. Hauppauge: Nova Science Publishers; 2011. p. 293–301.

73. Takei-Kumagai N, Lee S, Matsuzaki H, Hayashi H, Maeda M, Nishimura Y, Otsuki T. Silica, immunological effects. In: Uversky VN, Kretsinger RH, Permyakov EA, editors. Encyclopedia of metalloproteins. New York: Springer Science+Business Media; 2013. p. 1956–71.

74. Lee S, Maeda M, Hayashi H, Matsuzaki H, Kumagai-Takei N, Nishimura Y. Otsuki Immunostimulation by silica particles and the development of autoimmune dysregulation. In: Guy Huynh Thien D, editor. Immune response activation. Rijeka: InTech publisher; 2014. p. 249–65.

Chapter 3
Engineered Nanomaterials and Occupational Allergy

Claudia Petrarca, Luca Di Giampaolo, Paola Pedata, Sara Cortese, and Mario Di Gioacchino

Abstract The expanding demand for highly performing devices and products has prompted the development of innovative nanosized materials. This fact, along with the uncertain efficacy of protective equipment available for the nanosized particles, poses concern about the risk of becoming sensitised in the occupational setting. Actually, such a phenomenon can also affect the general population given the unavoidable environmental contamination. At the same time, studies on the physiopathology of the allergy demonstrated that the lack of prevention and treatment can result in invalidating diseases that, in case of professional aetiology, might imply removal from job and compensation. The potential role of nanomaterials in the development and exacerbation of occupational allergy is being disclosed by recent

C. Petrarca (✉)
Immuntotoxicology and Allergy Unit & Occupational Biorepository,
Center of Excellence on Aging and Translational Medicine (CeSI-MeT), "G. D'Annunzio"
University Foundation, Chieti, Italy
e-mail: c.petrarca@unich.it

L. Di Giampaolo
Department of Medical Oral and Biotechnological Science, G. d'Annunzio University,
Chieti, Italy

P. Pedata
Department of Experimental Medicine, Section of Hygiene, Occupational Medicine and
Forensic Medicine, Second University of Naples, Naples, Italy

S. Cortese
Department of Medicine and Science of Aging, G. d'Annunzio University, Chieti, Italy

M. Di Gioacchino
Immuntotoxicology and Allergy Unit & Occupational Biorepository,
Center of Excellence on Aging and Translational Medicine (CeSI-MeT), "G. D'Annunzio"
University Foundation, Chieti, Italy

Department of Medicine and Science of Aging, G. d'Annunzio University, Chieti, Italy

© Springer Science+Business Media Singapore 2017
T. Otsuki et al. (eds.), *Allergy and Immunotoxicology in Occupational Health*,
Current Topics in Environmental Health and Preventive Medicine,
DOI 10.1007/978-981-10-0351-6_3

experimental investigations in cellular and animal models. Moreover, first emerging data from professional human exposure are adding new information to the complex puzzled picture of nanotoxicology.

Most importantly, a deeper knowledge on the role of nanomaterials in the aetiology of the allergic diseases will allow the implementation of risk assessment and preventive measures for nanosafety at the workplace. Original articles retrieved from PubMed and Google searches using the keywords, occupational, exposure, workers, nanoparticles, nanomaterials, allergy as well as congress proceedings, institutional reports and unpublished data from research laboratories involved in this field have been considered as a source of updated information to write this chapter.

Keywords Nanomaterials • Nanoparticles • Allergy • Occupational • Workers • Nanosafety • Health surveillance • Research

3.1 Introduction

Nowadays, allergic diseases affect more than one third of the word population. Amongst them, those with an occupational cause appear to be common and are increasing, as observed by a recent esteem of the worldwide prevalence ranging from 5 to 15 % [1, 2]. Asthma, rhinitis, conjunctivitis, urticaria and contact dermatitis can be allergic, triggered by occupational factors such as high and low molecular weight substances acting as complete antigens or haptens. Moreover, according to epidemiological and experimental evidences, respiratory allergy could induce an inflammatory process leading to pulmonary function decline, which is a highly threatening condition exacerbated by the persistence of occupational allergen exposure [3]. Engineered nanomaterials, intentionally designed with specific properties for a wide range of technological applications, might contribute to the increasing prevalence of those diseases amongst workers [4]. In fact, due to the rapid advancements in this field, workers from nanotech industries and research laboratories might be exposed to these new materials. In this regard, occupational health risks associated with nanomaterials are still undefined, and little information is available on main exposure routes, potential exposure levels and toxicity [5]. The professional exposure is likely to occur during the post-production phase, while the reaction chamber is opened, when the product is handled, or during the cleanout procedures [6]. At research workplaces, the handling of dry powders of nanoparticles can generate airborne nanoparticles able to reach the breathing zone [7]. A recent Dutch study addresses many different categories of workers being potentially at risk of exposure to nanomaterials in that country [8].

So far, it has been difficult to assess the level of environmental contamination and the internal dose in exposed workers due to recent introduction of measure devices, still under evaluation, and lack of bioassays. It is well established, for instance, that aggregates and agglomerates, rather than solitaire nanoparticles, are the main components of a nano-substance within a fluid mean [9], which result difficult to split apart because of the shape and electrostatic charge. Therefore, these "multi-nanoparticle" entities are difficult to assess by the current measurement devices, nor it is possible to establish to which extent they can break up into smaller units in the lung fluid [10]. Generally, as we also do in this chapter, the term "nanoparticles" (NPs) is used to describe all the forms.

The assessment of the exposure level to NPs is made even more difficult for the copresence of other particles of different types, giving a background signal and the possible temporal changes in concentration [6].

An even more complex scenario comes from the fact that airborne chemicals can be adsorbed onto (nano)particles and gain new bioactive functions, as for the immunomodulatory effects characterising PM 0.5 (which include NPs) in industrial and traffic-influenced urban areas [11].

Nevertheless, some data are emerging on NP detection in biological matrixes of exposed workers. For instance, airborne titanium dioxide NPs were found in 40% of pre-shift samples and 70% of the post-shift samples of exhaled breath condensate of production workers, indicating the persistence of NPs; moreover, 10% of the post-shift urine samples contained NPs, confirming their translocation through the body [12]. It is well established that NPs can enter the human body upon exposure through inhalation, ingestion and absorption through the skin and reach tissues and cells [13]. Then, NPs can be included within exosomes, a sort of Trojan horse that allows them to spread from the capturing cells (macrophages and epithelial or endothelial cells) into the bloodstream and other cell types and tissues [14]; for metal-based NPs, there can be release of ions [15]. The case of cobalt is emblematic since NPs made of this metal rapidly release ions (Co^{2+}) in culture medium that are the true mediators of the observed toxic effects of cobalt NPs on 3T3 fibroblasts [16]. Ion-mediated effects of NPs have been described also for zinc oxide NPs influencing the cellular processes in macrophages [17]. Other interesting examples of NP dissolution are reported by Freitas and coworkers [18] for silver NPs of various sizes (10–40 nm) releasing ionic silver [Ag(I)] when dissolved alone in aqueous solution or mixed with copper ions [Cu(II)] or proteins and upon reaction with the metalloproteinase Cu(II) azurin. Particle dissolution is a similar mechanism also for the low toxicity and biopersistence in the lung of inhaled (50 mg·ml−1) barium sulphate NPs [19]. The release of ions from nickel sulphate NPs (nanoballs) is advantageously used for patch testing of nickel allergy [19]. The size [20], the aggregation tendency [21] and the capacity to form complexes with proteins (protein corona) [19, 22] contribute to determine the biological impact of NPs. For instance, BALB/c 3T3 fibroblasts undergo a higher degree of cell death when exposed to cobalt NPs rather than microparticles and ions [Co(II)] [16, 23], whereas only micro- and nanoparticles have morphological transforming potential [23]. Another study regarding the effect of cobalt NPs on gene expression indicates that innate immunity and apoptosis are influenced, whereas microparticles and ions affect different functional pathways [24].

Epidemiological data show that allergic reactions towards palladium, as contact dermatitis, are increased in the last decades in people living in urban settings where ultrafine particles (UFPs), including NPs of platinum group metals (GPE) and carbon, are released in the environment [25, 26].

Thus, are there scientific evidences supporting the role of nanosized material in the development and/or exacerbation of allergic diseases? Are there contacts or dermal sensitisers amongst nanomaterials? What are the possible mechanisms through which a pathological outcome might derive from professional exposure?

The aim of this chapter is to describe the recent findings about these issues and to analyse them in the perspective of occupational biosafety of nanowork.

3.2   Allergy-Related Biological Mechanisms of Nanomaterials In Vitro

The first event for a foreign antigen to evoke an immune response consists in the activation of the innate system cells. NPs are known to interact with these cells [27, 28], specifically devoted to getting rid of all non-self particulate matter entering the body. These defensive players, in particular macrophages and dendritic cells, detect and bind the NPs through molecular sensors adopted to identify bacterial and viral pathogens called Toll-like receptors (TLRs) [29], through which they can deliver signals in a size-dependent manner [30]. Such interaction can modify the activation status of these cells and their fundamental activities of phagocytosis and antigen presentation [31]. Moreover, following the interaction between NPs and the tissue-resident cells of the innate system, including neutrophils and mast cells, an inflammatory process is started that leads to the production of inflammatory mediators favouring vasodilation and chemotaxis [28]. The phagocytosis generates high levels of reactive oxygen species (ROS) produced to eliminate xeno-(nano)particles and linked to the pathogenetic potential of the NPs [28]. ROS induction is a critical step in the allergic response [32]. ROS can also be produced by the metal-based NPs of palladium and nickel for which a primary size-dependent catalytic mechanism has been described [33].

NPs may bind to antigenic proteins and induce conformational changes exposing cryptic epitopes (also used to obtain neo-allergens for therapeutic purposes) which, if exposed in humans, might trigger detrimental immune responses, including allergy [34].

A chemical substance can behave as a hapten able to form an immunogenic complex with a protein carrier inducing specific antibodies; in particular, given that crystals can only raise IgM, nanosized fullerene C60 is likely to act as such since it evokes the production of specific IgG [35].

Preliminary data regarding the in vitro responses of human immune cells challenged with NPs are coming up: LPS-activated lymphocytes from healthy subjects respond to the exposure to palladium NPs (5–10 nm) by internalising them in endocytic compartments and secreting high levels of IFN-γ (while inhibiting the tolerogenic cytokine IL-10) [36–38] suggesting a potential role in the Th1-mediated mechanism of delayed allergic reactions. IFN-γ release is also induced by multiwalled carbon nanotubes (MWCNTs) in mitogen-stimulated T cells from

Table 3.1 List of manufactured nanomaterials and their known allergy-relevant mechanisms of action based on in vitro studies

Manufactured nanomaterial		Cell model/species	Mechanisms/effects	References
Barium sulphate	BaSO$_4$		Ion release	[19, 22]
			Protein corona	
Carbon nanotubes, multiwalled (MWCNs)	C	Human T cells (mitogen-stimulated)/healthy and allergic humans	Induction of IFN-g (healthy subjects)	[29, 37]
			Inhibition of IL-5 (allergic subjects)	
Carbon nanotubes, single-walled (SWCNTs)	C		Toll-like receptor	[29, 38]
			Induction of IL-1	
Cobalt	Co	3T3 fibroblasts/	Ion release	[16, 19, 22]
		BALB/c mice	Protein corona	
Fullerene C60	C	–	Toll-like receptors	[29, 35]
			Apten	
Nickel oxide	Ni		ROS, catalytic activity	[31]
Palladium	Pd	Peripheral blood mononuclear cells/human, healthy	ROS, catalytic activity, induction of IFN-g	[31, 34–36]
Silver	Ag	–	Ion release	[18]
Titanium dioxide	TiO$_2$	Peripheral blood mononuclear cells/human	ROS, apoptosis	Personal data
Zinc oxide	ZnO	Macrophages	Ion release, impairment of cell function	[17]

healthy subjects, whereas they inhibit the allergen-induced release of IL-5 by peripheral blood mononuclear cells (PBMCs) from mite allergic patients [39]. Titanium dioxide NPs (7 nm, anatase) induce ROS increase in human PBMCs exposed to 25, 50 and 100 μg·ml^{-1} culture medium in a dose-dependent manner after 24 and 48 h incubation; in this system, ROS induction seems to be associated with the initiation of the programmed cell death (apoptosis) (personal unpublished data). Cellular response to carbon nanotube exposure involves upregulation of IL-1, participating to the intensification of the allergic inflammation [40]. Zinc oxide NPs, the most diffused NPs in consumer's goods, induce changes in the level of key proteins controlling cell survival and cancer (p53, Ras p21 and JNKs) in ex vivo lymphocytes isolated from lung tumours and chronic obstructive pulmonary disease (COPD) patients, but not in those from asthmatic subjects, compared to controls [41]. Allergy-relevant mechanisms of action and effects of the manufactured NPs based on in vitro findings are summarised in Table 3.1.

3.3   Allergy-Related Biological Mechanisms of Nanomaterials in Animal Models

It has been shown that NPs can cause specific immune reactions, immunosuppression and autoimmunity in animal models. Mouse and rat are considered well suited to mimic the basic immunological mechanisms of allergic sensitisation, atopic/contact dermatitis and asthma development. However, the validity to predict the sensitising and asthmogenic health risk for NP-exposed workers is not straightforward. In fact, the sensitivity against NPs seems to depend on the mouse strain [42]. Furthermore, the study design is crucial to obtain relevant data from animal models. In this regard, it seems that exposure to the test NPs should be done during the sensitisation and challenge phases. Moreover, studies should focus on the use of agglomerate/aggregate NPs. Even if not completely following such criteria and not using standardised NPs, a consistent amount of data are emerging from animal studies regarding allergy. The exposure route seems to be relevant for the observed findings: NPs cause inflammation of the lung if inhaled or instilled into the trachea or worsen the allergic airway inflammation and act as Th2 adjuvant following pulmonary exposure [43].

Some types of engineered nanomaterials induce immune responses in the lung; in particular, they appear to alter the allergen-induced eosinophilia [44] by modulating the balance between Th1, Th2 and Th17 cells [28].

Copper NPs are the most potent inducers of inflammation of the lung in a model of pulmonary bacterial infection sustained by neutrophils and inflammatory cytokines, an effect also caused by iron oxide NPs [45].

Adjuvant properties of NPs could have the undesirable effect of upholding allergic sensitisation. For instance, 3-day long subcutaneous or inhalant administration of carbon black NPs (22 and 39 nm) to transgenic mice (DO11.10) expressing the T cell receptor specific for the immunodominant peptide of ovalbumin (peptide 323–339) favours the sensitisation; in fact, secondary responses, induced in peptide-restimulated splenocytes in vitro, comprise Th2 cytokines (IL-4, IL-10 and IL-13) and reduced expression of the transcription factor Stat4, specific for Th1 cells. Notably, the authors find a relationship between the size of the particle and the magnitude of the effect. However, in this study, equal mass of the two types of NPs were compared implying that the total reactive surface was much higher for the smaller ones, accounting for the higher intensity of the observed responses. Nevertheless, carbon black NPs indeed showed a Th2 adjuvant effect in this animal model [46]. Also carbon nanofibres have IgE adjuvant capacity but are less potent than nanotubes in promoting allergic airway responses [47]. Engineered silica NPs act as adjuvants enhancing allergic airway disease in mice [48].

The direct implication of NPs in the exacerbation of pre-existing type I allergy has been shown in rats sensitised to ovalbumin. Intratracheally administered silicon dioxide NPs (nonspherical, 10–20 nm, 140–180 $m^2 \cdot g^{-1}$) induced increase of IL-4 in the lung tissue, airway remodelling and worsening of the respiratory parameters, with more pronounced effects at the highest dose (80 $\mu g \cdot ml^{-1}$) [49]. Notably, such adverse effects on lung function occur with or without ovalbumin immunisation [49]. These findings suggest that NPs may have a direct role in the development of bronchial asthma, not only as an exacerbating factor of a pre-existing allergic condition. Zinc oxide NPs provide an adjuvant effect to ovalbumin via a Th2 response [50], involving TLRs and Src signalling [51], and induce eosinophilic airway inflammation [44]. Moreover, these NPs (21 nm) do not affect oral tolerance [52].

A paradigm of the potential pro-allergic effect of nanoparticles comes from a study on cerium dioxide NPs, used for medical applications and also present as side products in the exhaust gas from diesel engines, able to generate multiple types of water-soluble NPs of concern for environmental and in vivo effects. Indeed, they are strongly suspected to promote allergic diseases since selectively taken up from alveolar macrophages and able to induce an inflammatory state [53].

Silver NPs have been associated with exacerbation of airway hyperactivity. Their role in the allergic sensitisation has been studied in experimental asthma induced by ovalbumin: the animals were exposed to 3.3 mg/ml NPs (33 nm) continuously inhaled; in both groups of healthy and sensitised mice, these NPs caused infiltration of neutrophils and lymphocytes in the airways (bronchocentric) and in the peritoneum at the sites of higher accrual; moreover, it induced elevation of mediators and effectors of the allergic response (total IgE, leukotriene E4 (LTE4), Th2 cells, IL-13 and oxidative stress) [54] and significant increase in allergen-specific IgE [55]. This same detrimental effect on the allergic airways was associated with altered VEGF signalling pathway and mucus hypersecretion [56]. Low-dose intratracheal instillation (0.2 mg per rat) of aggregates of nickel oxide NPs (26 nm) induces a transient increase in chemokines associated with relentless lung inflammation and in the expression of cytokines involved in allergy inflammation and fibrosis [57].

The case of iron oxide NPs is very interesting because the allergic response is suppressed or enhanced depending on the particle dose: in fact, iron oxide NPs intratracheally administered before and during ovalbumin sensitisation significantly inhibit the allergen-specific Th2 immune response at the two highest doses (4×250, 4×500 μg per mouse), whereas the lowest dose (4×100 μg per mouse) promotes the allergic response [58].

It is worth pointing out also that dermal exposure to combination of agglomerates of silica NPs and mite allergens induced an IgE-biased immune response and an increased sensitivity to anaphylaxis in not pre-sensitised mice [59].

Titanium dioxide NPs, the most produced amongst nanomaterials, are regarded as relatively nontoxic at the concentration levels of the occupational environments [60]. However, studies on inhalation exposure found this type of NPs to alter the inflammatory response in asthmatic mice [61]; moreover, they aggravate atopic dermatitis (AD)-like skin lesions in mice [62]. Lung injury-inducing high doses (32 mg·kg^{-1} twice a week for 4 weeks) of titanium dioxide NPs are not associated with significant changes of IL-4 in the lung, ruling out the involvement of an allergic reaction in the mechanism of damage [63]. Route-dependent immune effects are observed following exposure to titanium dioxide-NP immune effects [64]. Also the sensitisation status seems to determine different outcomes: ovalbumin-induced allergic pulmonary inflammation characterised by eosinophil infiltration in the lung and IL-4 is reduced upon inhalation of (agglomerated) titanium dioxide NPs (32 mg/ml for 6 and 42 h post-sensitisation) in asthmatic rats [65]; in non-sensitised rats, TiO_2 NPs (75 % anatase, 25 % rutile, 21 nm, aggregates of 200 nm and 2 μm, 5 mg·kg^{-1}) intratracheally instilled once provoke acute airway inflammation with transitory IL-4 production, replaced by a durable Th1 response [22]. In a mouse model, instead, the same component instilled at 5–50 mg·kg^{-1} (150 μm aggregate mean size) induced a Th2-mediated chronic inflammation, evidencing a species-related bias of the immune response [66].

Polystyrene NP application to atopic dermatitis-like skin lesions (related to mite allergen) induces local size-dependent increase of protein levels of IL-4 and various chemokine ligands for monocytes and macrophages recruitment [67], whereas, on normal skin, it induces sensitisation [68]. In the same AD (atopic dermatitis), an aggravation of the pathological condition is induced size dependently by amorphous silica NPs upon intradermal injection [69].

NPs of nickel oxide (NiO) and cobalt oxide (Co_3O_4) induce lung-delayed hypersensitivity-like responses in mice [70], whereas hydroxyapatite NPs do not produce any effect in the guinea pig model of this pathology [71]. Allergy-relevant mechanisms of action and effects of the manufactured NPs based on in vivo findings are summarised in Table 3.2.

Interestingly, relevant NPs in the field of advanced technologies, such as silver NPs and fullerene C60, own intrinsic capacity useful to control the allergic reactions; for instance, fullerene C60 was found to prevent the histamine release in a mast cell-dependent anaphylaxis model [72], and silver NPs (5 nm) reduce hyper-reactivity in a murine model of airway allergic inflammation, perhaps due to its antioxidant and anti-inflammatory activities [73]. Topically applied zinc oxide NPs (ZnO) suppress allergen-induced skin inflammation but induce vigorous IgE production in the atopic dermatitis mouse model [17].

3.4 Occupational Allergic Diseases with Potential Nanomaterial Aetiology

Taking into account the global experimental information gathered so far on the biological impact of nanomaterials, for exposed workers, the risk of developing nanoparticle-exposure associated pathologies cannot be totally ruled out, as well as exacerbating pre-existing pathologies. Moreover, it is conceivable that adverse health effects may especially develop in hypersensitive populations, such as individuals with respiratory diseases (Fig. 3.1). Whatever form and chemical species they acquire inside the body, engineered nanomaterials can induce oxidative stress responsible for lung diseases [74] attributable to their particulate physical form. Pleural effusion, pulmonary fibrosis and granuloma can be related to exposure to NPs [75]. The possibility of aggravation of chemically induced occupational asthma in the presence of NP exposure is suggested by recent findings showing that a very

Table 3.2 List of principal manufactured nanomaterials with high industrial burden and mechanisms favouring allergic diseases triggered by exposure described in animal studies

Nanomaterial	Formula	Production and usage sectors	Animal model	Exposure route	Mechanism	Biological/pathological outcome	References
Cerium dioxide	CeO_2	Medical applications	CD-1 mouse	Intratracheal	Release of water-soluble nanoparticles	Selective uptake by alveolar macrophages	[53]
					Pro-inflammatory		
Cobalt oxide	Co_3O_4	Sensors, energy, drug delivery	Healthy rats	Lung instillation	Apten	Delayed-time hypersensitivity	[70]
Copper	Cu	Electrical, engineering, transport, building and construction	Pulmonary bacterial infection in mice	Inhalant	Pro-inflammatory	Strong lung inflammation sustained by neutrophils and inflammatory cytokines	[45]
Carbon black	C	Tyres, printer toner, dyes for leather or textiles, cosmetics	Transgenic mice (OVA-specific T cell receptor)	Intratracheal	Th2 adjuvant	IL-4, IL-10 and IL-13	[46]
				Subcutaneous		Th1-specific Stat 4 transcription factor	
Carbon nanofibres	C	Power, wind energy, aeronautical, sports, construction, chemical, automotive	Healthy mice	Intratracheal	IgE adjuvant	Allergic airway disease	[47]
Iron oxide	FeO	Glass, paints, coatings, automotive	Healthy mice	Intratracheal	Neutrophil, inflammatory cytokines	Lung inflammation	[45, 58]
Nickel oxide	NiO	Microelectronics, aerospace materials, batteries, electrochromic coatings and materials	Healthy rats	Intratracheal	Pro-inflammatory	Th2 cytokines	[57, 70]
				0.2 mg per rat (low)		chemokines	
						Fibrosis	
						Sustained lung inflammation	
						Delayed-time hypersensitivity	

(continued)

Table 3.2 (continued)

Nanomaterial	Formula	Production and usage sectors	Animal model	Exposure route	Mechanism	Biological/pathological outcome	References
Polystyrene	$(C_8H_8)_n$	Atopic dermatitis mouse model	Healthy mice	On skin lesion	Pro-inflammatory	Site-dependent IL-4, chemokines	[67, 68]
				On normal skin		Sensitisation	
Silicon dioxide	SiO_2	Concrete, plastics, synthetic materials	OVA-sensitised rats	Intratracheal 140–180 $m^2 \cdot g^{-1}$	Adjuvant of type I allergy	Induction of IL-4	[48, 49, 59, 69]
			Healthy rats			Allergic airway disease (<u>only sensitised</u>)	
						Adverse effect on lung function	
Silver	Ag	Plastics, synthetic materials	OVA-sensitised mice	Inhalant 7 days continuously	Th2 adjuvant	Induction of IL-4, IL-13, total IgE, allergen-specific IgE, LTE-4, Th2 cells, neutrophils	[54–56]
						Oxidative stress	
						Exacerbation of airway hyperactivity	
						VEGF	
			Healthy mice	3.3 $mg \cdot m^{-3}$	Pro-inflammatory	Mucus hypersecretion	
Titanium dioxide	TiO_2	Cosmetics and paint	AD mouse model	Topical	ROS, apoptosis	Aggravation of AD	[22, 61–66]
			Healthy mice	Inhalant		Lung injury (IL-4 independent)	
			Healthy rats/mice	Intratracheal			
			OVA-sensitised mice			Th1 response/Th2-mediated inflammation	
Zinc oxide	ZnO	Cosmetics and paint	OVA-sensitised mice		Th2 adjuvant	Eosinophilic airway inflammation	[44, 50, 51]
			AD mouse model			Induction of IgE	

low dose (approx. 0.8 mg·kg^{-1}) of intrapulmonary gold or titanium dioxide NPs modulates a non-IgE-mediated asthma [76, 77] (Fig. 3.1). The pro-inflammatory activity shown by most nanomaterials makes plausible the hypothesis that the occupational exposure might provide stimuli able to trigger sarcoidosis-like illness (giant cell-like nodules), typically affecting individuals exposed to foreign antigens and to inorganic particulates and recognised and compensable as work-associated disease [78].

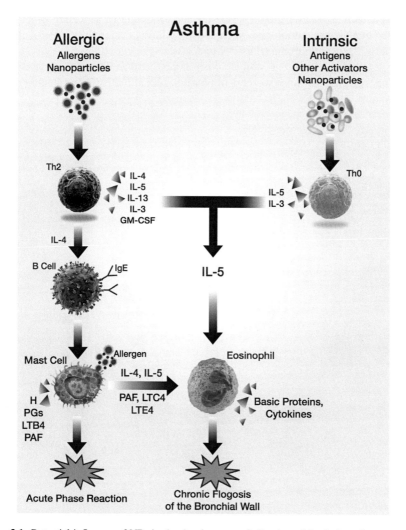

Fig. 3.1 Potential influence of NPs in the development of allergic and intrinsic asthma, as suggested by in vitro and in vivo findings. Pathways and molecules possibly affected by NPs activity are coloured in *red* (Modified from [89])

It is well known that occupational asthma may be caused by metals (e.g. cobalt, platinum, chromium, vanadium, nickel) and that sensitisation to the professional agent is one of the known aetiopathogenetic mechanisms triggering this immuno-logically mediated disease. It has been found that also nanosized metals own pro-sensitising effects in vitro and in vivo, suggesting a potential role in the development of this life-threatening professional disease (Fig. 3.1). The most challenging of them regards the possibility of acting as such, as aptens or as released ions once inside the body.

Even more concerning, a role cannot be excluded for nanoparticles in the exacerbation of pre-existing eosinophil-mediated allergic diseases of nonoccupational aetiology, such as rhinitis, atopic dermatitis and food allergy, as well as other Th2-mediated nonallergic pathologies, such as aspergillosis, eosinophilic gastroenteritis and Churg-Strauss syndrome (Figs. 3.1 and 3.2).

Pro-sensitising effects, as well as other unpredictable immunological effects, might be worrying for those workers of pharmaceutical industries producing nano-

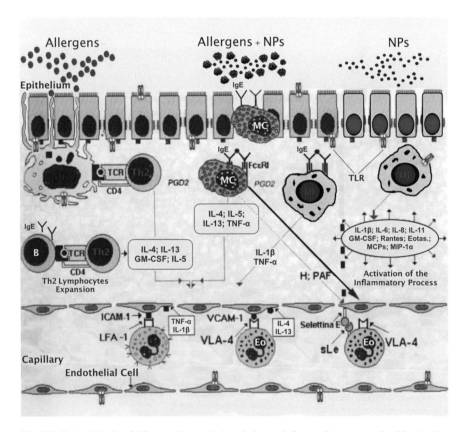

Fig. 3.2 Potential role of NPs on allergen-induced airway inflammation, as sustained by in vitro and in vivo data. Cell types, pathways and molecular mediators emerging to be influenced by NPs are coloured in *red* (Modified from [89])

vaccines made of NPs loaded with immunogenic proteins to be used for immunotherapy or functionalised on the surface to generate immunoactivating compounds for anticancer therapy. Several anti-allergy nanovaccines have been designed so far with the purpose of switching off the detrimental immune response towards an allergen. They consist of porous and/or polymeric substances (PLGA, dextran, silica) with adjuvant activity (either intrinsic or conferred by LPS) that are loaded [17, 79, 80] or agglomerated [81] with the therapeutic allergen. In vitro and in vivo experimental testing of these products has been carried out recently. The results suggest beneficial effects of these nanovaccines in allergic asthma and atopic dermatitis model that appear to rely on the potentiated adjuvancy given by the NP component. In particular, the treatment with PLGA profilin modifies the Th2/Th1 cytokine balance and inhibits the differentiation of eosinophils [79]; dextran-NP ovalbumin activates the antigen-presenting cells and induces potent immunomodulation and proliferative responses of allergen-specific T cells (experimentally grafted in mice) [80]. Moreover, zinc oxide NPs, designed for local treatment of atopic dermatitis, are able to suppress allergen-induced skin inflammation in the mouse model of this disease but also to induce strong IgE production [17].

A very high rate of immunoactivation of bone marrow-derived dendritic cells (MDDCs) and T cells is achieved experimentally by exposing these cells to porous silicon nanoplatforms designed for immunotherapy, with dependency on surface chemistry [82].

3.5 Nanoparticle Sensitising Effects in Humans

Data on the effects of occupational exposure to NPs are very limited. In fact, their ability to induce sensitisation has been investigated for a chronic nonoccupational exposure due to hip replacement with cobalt-chromium-coated polyethylene NP-based prosthesis, characterised by strong metal ion release. There was a significant increase of the two metals in the urine of the subjects who had received this type of prosthesis, compared with those who had received the standard non-NP type; however, no relative increase of metal allergy was observed, with a follow-up of 5 years after surgery [83]. Even though this study does not attribute to in vivo NPs with a higher sensitising potential compared to non-nanomaterials, this conclusion is made on a limited number of subjects and a short time of observation, while the long-term effects are not predictable [83]. Recently, a first human study of a systemically ingested silver-NP product [84] has been carried out. Also in this case, silver was present in serum supposed to be mostly in the ionic form, since after 14 days no evidence was found of intact silver NPs absorbed through the human digestive tract or attached to blood components. Moreover, no clinically significant changes in metabolic, haematologic, urine and physical findings, sputum morphology and/or imaging changes were observed. Hence, even for exposed workers, ion released from metal NPs could represent a potential allergic/health threat.

Human data are available from volunteers exposed, in research settings, to diesel exhaust particulate (DEP) containing NPs (at $>10^6$ particles·cm^{-3}, far exceeding the worst-case exposure for workers) for whom elevated exposures have been associated with temporary lung and systemic inflammation, thrombogenesis, vascular function and brain activity with no evidence of a unique toxicity for NPs, as compared to other particles, and not supporting acute toxicity of NPs (at least within DEP) by virtue of their exclusive nanosize [85].

Although no prospective studies have still been conducted, several case reports are already available.

In 2009, seven healthy women experienced short breath and pleural effusions after 5–13 months of occupational exposure to polyacrylate NPs. These symptoms were associated with the presence of NPs in cells and chest fluid along with lung inflammation fibrosis and granuloma of the pleura. However, there were no findings of allergic responses or other immunological impairments [75].

A 22-year-old student involved in work leading to synthesis of dendrimers (nanosized particles used as drug carriers) developed contact dermatitis (erythema multiforme-like) on his hands that progressed to involve other areas of the body. Despite treatment with topical steroids and antihistamines, it required hospitalisation for more than 3 weeks. However, professional re-exposure caused recurrence of the symptoms [86].

In 2014, a case report was published about a healthy 26-year-old nonsmoking female working in an industry producing metallic inks who was assigned the task of weighting out repeatedly 1–2 g of dry nickel-NP (20 nm, 40–60 m^2·g^{-1}) powder on the laboratory bench without wearing any personal protection. Then, she developed throat congestion with postnasal drip and flushing of the face; concomitantly, she manifested skin reactions to earrings and belt buckle, never observed before. The patch test reacted positively to nickel sulphate in the standard patch testing [87].

The conclusions of a recent epidemiologic questionnaire-based study on workers handling various types of NPs aiming at highlighting the link between the levels of exposure and symptoms revealed sneezing as the only significant work-related effect and allergic dermatitis as the only disease significantly worsened [88].

3.6   Discussion

It is demanding to assess whether nanomaterials can act as inducing and promoting risk factors to safely develop nanotechnology and nanowork. This chapter represents an attempt to collect up-to-date findings and rationalise them for such purpose, giving special focus on nanoparticle-related allergy risk. It is clear that data collected so far come from heterogeneous experimental studies that are affected by a bias due to the poor characterisation of nanomatter once it reaches the human biological matrixes. In fact, although a precise characterisation can be obtained for the manufactured nanomaterial products, upon interaction of nanoparticles with the organism, the newly acquired properties are virtually not predictable and rather complex to measure (by using radioactive nanomaterials, for instance). This makes it difficult to obtain an unequivocal assessment of a cause-effect relationship. Moreover, in order to achieve an experimental result, high doses and short time of exposure are applied; whereas the level of contamination is expected to be rather low in the workplace for a chronic mode of exposure.

Lack of human data for the potential toxicity is due to two main reasons: challenge studies are not feasible in man and, in the environment, NPs are contaminated with other numerous substances that modulate their activity. For this reason, the workplace could represent an outstanding experimental setting because the level and the condition of exposure are well measurable; moreover, the health surveillance programme might provide the follow-up data to identify the onset and progression of any possible diseases. Researchers should take advantage of this circumstance to carry out studies on pathogenetic mechanisms.

Being one of the epidemics of the century and one of the most prevalent diseases in workers, allergy should be logical to carefully evaluate the risk induced by NPs in exposed workers. Available data provide the justification for this attention. There are studies (few) sustaining that NP exposure is associated with the appearance of allergic pathologies, either cutaneous or IgE mediated, supported by in vitro and in animal findings showing that various NPs are able to induce immunological modifications typical of allergy. By combining health surveillance and scientific research, it will be possible to assess nanomaterial effects on human health and prompt the safe and sustainable production and use of nanomaterials.

Acknowledgements We thank Dr Flavia Carpiniello for the assistance in the revision of the English language and the graphical aid.

References

1. Slavin R. Occupational rhinitis. Immunol Allergy Clin N Am. 1992;12:769.
2. Slavin RG. Update on occupational rhinitis and asthma. Allergy Asthma Proc 31:437–43. doi:10.2500/aap.2010.31.3379.
3. Di Giampaolo L, Cavallucci E, Braga M, Renzetti A, Schiavone C, Quecchia C, et al. The persistence of allergen exposure favors pulmonary function decline in workers with allergic occupational asthma. Int Arch Occup Environ Health. 2012;85:181–8. doi:10.1007/s00420-011-0653-4.
4. ISO/TR 27628. Workplace atmospheres. Ultrafine, nanoparticle and nano-structured aerosols. Inhalation exposure characterization and assessment, 2007. n.d.
5. http://www.cdc.gov/niosh/topics/nanotech/. n.d.
6. Kazula S, Balderhaar J, Orthen B, Onnhert B, Jankoswka E, Rosell MG, Tanarro C, Tejeodor JZA. Literature review – workplace exposure to nanoparticles. OSHA – Eur Agency Saf Heal Work. n.d.; https://os.
7. Tsai, SJ, Ada, E, Ellenbecker M. Airborne nanoparticle exposures associated with the manual handling of nanoaluminia in fume hood. 3rd international symposium on nanotechnology, occupational environmental health, Taipei, Taiwan, 2007.

42   C. Petrarca et al.

8. Bekker C, Brouwer DH, Tielemans E, Pronk A. Industrial production and professional application of manufactured nanomaterials-enabled end products in Dutch industries: potential for exposure. Ann Occup Hyg. 2013;57:314–27. doi:10.1093/annhyg/mes072.

9. Tiede K, Tear SP, David H, Boxall ABA. Imaging of engineered nanoparticles and their aggregates under fully liquid conditions in environmental matrices. Water Res. 2009;43:3335–43. doi:10.1016/j.watres.2009.04.045.

10. Fujitani Y, Kobayashi T, Arashidani K, Kunugita N, Suemura K. Measurement of the physical properties of aerosols in a fullerene factory for inhalation exposure assessment. J Occup Environ Hyg. 2008;5:380–9. doi:10.1080/15459620802050053.

11. Wichmann G, Franck U, Herbarth O, Rehwagen M, Dietz A, Massolo L, et al. Different immunomodulatory effects associated with sub-micrometer particles in ambient air from rural, urban and industrial areas. Toxicology. 2009;257:127–36. doi:10.1016/j.tox.2008.12.024.

12. Pelclova D, Barosova H, Kukutschova J, Zdimal V, Navratil T, Fenclova Z, et al. Raman microspectroscopy of exhaled breath condensate and urine in workers exposed to fine and nano TiO_2 particles: a cross-sectional study. J Breath Res. 2015;9:036008. doi:10.1088/1752-7155/9/3/036008.

13. Petrarca C, Clemente E, Di Giampaolo L, Mariani-Costantini R, Leopold K, Schindl R, et al. Palladium nanoparticles induce disturbances in cell cycle entry and progression of peripheral blood mononuclear cells: paramount role of ions. J Immunol Res. 2014;2014:295092. doi:10.1155/2014/295092.

14. Zhu M, Li Y, Shi J, Feng W, Nie G, Zhao Y. Exosomes as extrapulmonary signaling conveyors for nanoparticle-induced systemic immune activation. Small. 2012;8:404–12. doi:10.1002/smll.201101708.

15. Horev-Azaria L, Kirkpatrick CJ, Korenstein R, Marche PN, Maimon O, Ponti J, et al. Predictive toxicology of cobalt nanoparticles and ions: comparative *in vitro* study of different cellular models using methods of knowledge discovery from data. Toxicol Sci. 2011;122:489–501. doi:10.1093/toxsci/kfr124.

16. Sabbioni E, Fortaner S, Farina M, Del Torchio R, Petrarca C, Bernardini G, et al. Interaction with culture medium components, cellular uptake and intracellular distribution of cobalt nanoparticles, microparticles and ions in Balb/3T3 mouse fibroblasts. Nanotoxicology. 2014;8:88–99. doi:10.3109/17435390.2012.752051.

17. Ilves M, Palomäki J, Vippola M, Lehto M, Savolainen K, Savinko T, et al. Topically applied ZnO nanoparticles suppress allergen induced skin inflammation but induce vigorous IgE production in the atopic dermatitis mouse model. Part Fibre Toxicol. 2014;11:38. doi:10.1186/s12989-014-0038-4.

18. Freitas DN, Martinolich AJ, Amaris ZN, Wheeler KE. Beyond the passive interactions at the nano-bio interface: evidence of Cu metalloprotein-driven oxidative dissolution of silver nanoparticles. J Nanobiotechnol. 2016;14:7. doi:10.1186/s12951-016-0160-6.

19. Sugiyama T, Uo M, Wada T, Hongo T, Omagari D, Komiyama K, et al. Novel metal allergy patch test using metal nanoballs. J Nanobiotechnol. 2014;12:51. doi:10.1186/s12951-014-0051-7.

20. Liu W, Wu Y, Wang C, Li HC, Wang T, Liao CY, et al. Impact of silver nanoparticles on human cells: effect of particle size. Nanotoxicology. 2010;4:319–30. doi:10.3109/17435390.2010.483745.

21. Nel A, Xia T, Mädler L, Li N. Toxic potential of materials at the nanolevel. Science. 2006;311:622–7. doi:10.1126/science.1114397.

22. Gustafsson Å, Lindstedt E, Elfsmark LS, Bucht A. Lung exposure of titanium dioxide nanoparticles induces innate immune activation and long-lasting lymphocyte response in the Dark Agouti rat. J Immunotoxicol. 2011;8:111–21. doi:10.3109/1547691X.2010.546382.

23. Sabbioni E, Fortaner S, Farina M, Del Torchio R, Olivato I, Petrarca C, et al. Cytotoxicity and morphological transforming potential of cobalt nanoparticles, microparticles and ions in Balb/3T3 mouse fibroblasts: an *in vitro* model. Nanotoxicology. 2014;8:455–64. doi:10.3109/17435390.2013.796538.

24. Perconti S, Aceto GM, Verginelli F, Napolitano F, Petrarca C, Bernardini G, et al. Distinctive gene expression profiles in Balb/3T3 cells exposed to low dose cobalt nanoparticles, microparticles and ions: potential nanotoxicological relevance. J Biol Regul Homeost Agents. 2013;27:443–54.

25. Santucci B, Valenzano C, de Rocco M, Cristaudo A. Platinum in the environment: frequency of reactions to platinum-group elements in patients with dermatitis and urticaria. Contact Dermatitis. 2000;43:333–8.

26. Muris J, Goossens A, Gonçalo M, Bircher AJ, Giménez-Arnau A, Foti C, et al. Sensitization to palladium and nickel in Europe and the relationship with oral disease and dental alloys. Contact Dermatitis. 2015;72:286–96. doi:10.1111/cod.12327.

27. Petrarca C, Clemente E, Amato V, Pedata P, Sabbioni E, Bernardini G, et al. Engineered metal based nanoparticles and innate immunity. Clin Mol Allergy. 2015;13:13. doi:10.1186/s12948-015-0020-1.

28. Thompson EA, Sayers BC, Glista-Baker EE, Shipkowski KA, Taylor AJ, Bonner JC. Innate immune responses to nanoparticle exposure in the lung. J Environ Immunol Toxicol 1:150–6. doi:10.7178/jeit.23.

29. Turabekova M, Rasulev B, Theodore M, Jackman J, Leszczynska D, Leszczynski J. Immunotoxicity of nanoparticles: a computational study suggests that CNTs and C60 fullerenes might be recognized as pathogens by Toll-like receptors. Nanoscale. 2014;6:3488–95. doi:10.1039/c3nr05772k.

30. Tsai C-Y, Lu S-L, Hu C-W, Yeh C-S, Lee G-B, Lei H-Y. Size-dependent attenuation of TLR9 signaling by gold nanoparticles in macrophages. J Immunol. 2012;188:68–76. doi:10.4049/jimmunol.1100344.

31. Kodali V, Littke MH, Tilton SC, Teeguarden JG, Shi L, Frevert CW, et al. Dysregulation of macrophage activation profiles by engineered nanoparticles. ACS Nano. 2013;7:6997–7010. doi:10.1021/nn402145t.

32. Boldogh I, Bacsi A, Choudhury BK, Dharajiya N, Alam R, Hazra TK, et al. ROS generated by pollen NADPH oxidase provide a signal that augments antigen-induced allergic airway inflammation. J Clin Invest. 2005;115:2169–79. doi:10.1172/JCI24422.

33. Neubauer N, Palomaeki J, Karisola P, Alenius H, Kasper G. Size-dependent ROS production by palladium and nickel nanoparticles in cellular and acellular environments – an indication for the catalytic nature of their interactions. Nanotoxicology. 2015:1–8. doi:10.3109/1743539 0.2015.1019585.

34. Tsuzuky T, editor. Nanotechnology commercialization. CRC Press Taylor & Francis Group; 2013. Boca Raton, Florida, USA.

35. Izhaky D, Pecht I. What else can the immune system recognize? Proc Natl Acad Sci U S A. 1998;95:11509–10.

36. Petrarca C, Perrone A, Verna N, Verginelli F, Ponti J, Sabbioni E, et al. Cobalt nano-particles modulate cytokine in vitro release by human mononuclear cells mimicking autoimmune disease. Int J Immunopathol Pharmacol. 2006;19:11–4.

37. Boscolo P, Bellante V, Leopold K, Maier M, Di Giampaolo L, Antonucci A, et al. Effects of palladium nanoparticles on the cytokine release from peripheral blood mononuclear cells of non-atopic women. J Biol Regul Homeost Agents. 2010;24:207–14.

38. Di Gioacchino M, Petrarca C, Lazzarin F, Di Giampaolo L, Sabbioni E, Boscolo P, et al. Immunotoxicity of nanoparticles. Int J Immunopathol Pharmacol. 2011;24:65S–71.

39. Laverny G, Casset A, Purohit A, Schaeffer E, Spiegelhalter C, de Blay F, et al. Immunomodulatory properties of multi-walled carbon nanotubes in peripheral blood mononuclear cells from healthy subjects and allergic patients. Toxicol Lett. 2013;217:91–101. doi:10.1016/j.toxlet.2012.12.008.

40. Arnoldussen YJ, Skogstad A, Skaug V, Kasem M, Haugen A, Benker N, et al. Involvement of IL-1 genes in the cellular responses to carbon nanotube exposure. Cytokine. 2015;73:128–37. doi:10.1016/j.cyto.2015.01.032.

41. Kumar A, Najafzadeh M, Jacob BK, Dhawan A, Anderson D. Zinc oxide nanoparticles affect the expression of p53, Ras p21 and JNKs: an ex vivo/*in vitro* exposure study in respiratory disease patients. Mutagenesis. 2015;30:237–45. doi:10.1093/mutage/geu064.

42. Inoue K-I, Takano H. The effect of nanoparticles on airway allergy in mice. Eur Respir J. 2011;37:1300–1. doi:10.1183/09031936.00027211.

43. Inoue K. Promoting effects of nanoparticles/materials on sensitive lung inflammatory diseases. Environ Health Prev Med. 2011;16:139–43. doi:10.1007/s12199-010-0177-7.

44. Huang K-L, Lee Y-H, Chen H-I, Liao H-S, Chiang B-L, Cheng T-J. Zinc oxide nanoparticles induce eosinophilic airway inflammation in mice. J Hazard Mater. 2015;297:304–12. doi:10.1016/j.jhazmat.2015.05.023.

45. Kim JS, Adamcakova-Dodd A, O'Shaughnessy PT, Grassian VH, Thorne PS. Effects of copper nanoparticle exposure on host defense in a murine pulmonary infection model. Part Fibre Toxicol. 2011;8:29. doi:10.1186/1743-8977-8-29.

46. Lefebvre DE, Pearce B, Fine JH, Chomyshyn E, Ross N, Halappanavar S, et al. In vitro enhancement of mouse T helper 2 cell sensitization to ovalbumin allergen by carbon black nanoparticles. Toxicol Sci. 2014;138:322–32. doi:10.1093/toxsci/kfu010.

47. Nygaard UC, Samuelsen M, Marioara CD, Løvik M. Carbon nanofibers have IgE adjuvant capacity but are less potent than nanotubes in promoting allergic airway responses. Biomed Res Int. 2013;2013:476010. doi:10.1155/2013/476010.

48. Brandenberger C, Rowley NL, Jackson-Humbles DN, Zhang Q, Bramble LA, Lewandowski RP, et al. Engineered silica nanoparticles act as adjuvants to enhance allergic airway disease in mice. Part Fibre Toxicol. 2013;10:26. doi:10.1186/1743-8977-10-26.

49. Han B, Guo J, Abrahaley T, Qin L, Wang L, Zheng Y, et al. Adverse effect of nano-silicon dioxide on lung function of rats with or without ovalbumin immunization. PLoS ONE. 2011;6:e17236. doi:10.1371/journal.pone.0017236.

50. Roy R, Kumar S, Verma AK, Sharma A, Chaudhari BP, Tripathi A, et al. Zinc oxide nanoparticles provide an adjuvant effect to ovalbumin via a Th2 response in Balb/c mice. Int Immunol. 2014;26:159–72. doi:10.1093/intimm/dxt053.

51. Roy R, Kumar D, Sharma A, Gupta P, Chaudhari BP, Tripathi A, et al. ZnO nanoparticles induced adjuvant effect via toll-like receptors and Src signaling in Balb/c mice. Toxicol Lett. 2014;230:421–33. doi:10.1016/j.toxlet.2014.08.008.

52. Matsumura M, Takasu N, Nagata M, Nakamura K, Kawai M, Yoshino S. Effect of ultrafine zinc oxide (ZnO) nanoparticles on induction of oral tolerance in mice. J Immunotoxicol 7:232–7. doi:10.3109/1547691X.2010.487879.

53. Poma A, Ragnelli AM, de Lapuente J, Ramos D, Borras M, Aimola P, et al. In vivo inflammatory effects of ceria nanoparticles on CD-1 mouse: evaluation by hematological, histological, and TEM analysis. J Immunol Res. 2014;2014:361419. doi:10.1155/2014/361419.

54. Chuang H-C, Hsiao T-C, Wu C-K, Chang H-H, Lee C-H, Chang C-C, et al. Allergenicity and toxicology of inhaled silver nanoparticles in allergen-provocation mice models. Int J Nanomedicine. 2013;8:4495–506. doi:10.2147/IJN.S52239.

55. Su C-L, Chen T-T, Chang C-C, Chuang K-J, Wu C-K, Liu W-T, et al. Comparative proteomics of inhaled silver nanoparticles in healthy and allergen provoked mice. Int J Nanomedicine. 2013;8:2783–99. doi:10.2147/IJN.S46997.

56. Jang S, Park JW, Cha HR, Jung SY, Lee JE, Jung SS, et al. Silver nanoparticles modify VEGF signaling pathway and mucus hypersecretion in allergic airway inflammation. Int J Nanomedicine. 2012;7:1329–43. doi:10.2147/IJN.S27159.

57. Morimoto Y, Ogami A, Todoroki M, Yamamoto M, Murakami M, Hirohashi M, et al. Expression of inflammation-related cytokines following intratracheal instillation of nickel oxide nanoparticles. Nanotoxicology. 2010;4:161–76. doi:10.3109/17435390903518479.

58. Ban M, Langonné I, Huguet N, Guichard Y, Goutet M. Iron oxide particles modulate the ovalbumin-induced Th2 immune response in mice. Toxicol Lett. 2013;216:31–9. doi:10.1016/j.toxlet.2012.11.003.

59. Hirai T, Yoshioka Y, Takahashi H, Ichihashi K, Udaka A, Mori T, et al. Cutaneous exposure to agglomerates of silica nanoparticles and allergen results in IgE-biased immune response and increased sensitivity to anaphylaxis in mice. Part Fibre Toxicol. 2015;12:16. doi:10.1186/s12989-015-0095-3.
60. Lindenschmidt RC, Driscoll KE, Perkins MA, Higgins JM, Maurer JK, Belfiore KA. The comparison of a fibrogenic and two nonfibrogenic dusts by bronchoalveolar lavage. Toxicol Appl Pharmacol. 1990;102:268–81.
61. Jonasson S, Gustafsson A, Koch B, Bucht A. Inhalation exposure of nano-scaled titanium dioxide (TiO2) particles alters the inflammatory responses in asthmatic mice. Inhal Toxicol. 2013;25:179–91. doi:10.3109/08958378.2013.770939.
62. Yanagisawa R, Takano H, Inoue K-I, Koike E, Kamachi T, Sadakane K, et al. Titanium dioxide nanoparticles aggravate atopic dermatitis-like skin lesions in NC/Nga mice. Exp Biol Med (Maywood). 2009;234:314–22. doi:10.3181/0810-RM-304.
63. Chang X, Fu Y, Zhang Y, Tang M, Wang B. Effects of Th1 and Th2 cells balance in pulmonary injury induced by nano titanium dioxide. Environ Toxicol Pharmacol. 2013;37:275–83. doi:10.1016/j.etap.2013.12.001.
64. Auttachoat W, McLoughlin CE, White KL, Smith MJ. Route-dependent systemic and local immune effects following exposure to solutions prepared from titanium dioxide nanoparticles. J Immunotoxicol. 11:273–82. doi:10.3109/1547691X.2013.844750.
65. Scarino A, Noël A, Renzi PM, Cloutier Y, Vincent R, Truchon G, et al. Impact of emerging pollutants on pulmonary inflammation in asthmatic rats: ethanol vapors and agglomerated TiO2 nanoparticles. Inhal Toxicol. 2012;24:528–38. doi:10.3109/08958378.2012.696741.
66. Park E-J, Yoon J, Choi K, Yi J, Park K. Induction of chronic inflammation in mice treated with titanium dioxide nanoparticles by intratracheal instillation. Toxicology. 2009;260:37–46. doi:10.1016/j.tox.2009.03.005.
67. Yanagisawa R, Takano H, Inoue KI, Koike E, Sadakane K, Ichinose T. Size effects of polystyrene nanoparticles on atopic dermatitis like skin lesions in NC/NGA mice. Int J Immunopathol Pharmacol 23:131–41.
68. Park Y-H, Jeong SH, Yi SM, Choi BH, Kim Y-R, Kim I-K, et al. Analysis for the potential of polystyrene and TiO2 nanoparticles to induce skin irritation, phototoxicity, and sensitization. Toxicol in Vitro. 2011;25:1863–9. doi:10.1016/j.tiv.2011.05.022.
69. Hirai T, Yoshikawa T, Nabeshi H, Yoshida T, Tochigi S, Ichihashi K, et al. Amorphous silica nanoparticles size-dependently aggravate atopic dermatitis-like skin lesions following an intradermal injection. Part Fibre Toxicol. 2012;9:3. doi:10.1186/1743-8977-9-3.
70. Cho W-S, Duffin R, Bradley M, Megson IL, Macnee W, Howie SEM, et al. NiO and Co3O4 nanoparticles induce lung DTH-like responses and alveolar lipoproteinosis. Eur Respir J. 2012;39:546–57. doi:10.1183/09031936.00047111.
71. Geetha CS, Remya NS, Leji KB, Syama S, Reshma SC, Sreekanth PJ, et al. Cells-nano interactions and molecular toxicity after delayed hypersensitivity, in guinea pigs on exposure to hydroxyapatite nanoparticles. Colloids Surf B: Biointerfaces. 2013;112:204–12. doi:10.1016/j.colsurfb.2013.07.058.
72. Ryan JJ, Bateman HR, Stover A, Gomez G, Norton SK, Zhao W, et al. Fullerene nanomaterials inhibit the allergic response. J Immunol. 2007;179:665–72.
73. Park HS, Kim KH, Jang S, Park JW, Cha HR, Lee JE, et al. Attenuation of allergic airway inflammation and hyperresponsiveness in a murine model of asthma by silver nanoparticles. Int J Nanomedicine. 2010;5:505–15.
74. Li N, Xia T, Nel AE. The role of oxidative stress in ambient particulate matter-induced lung diseases and its implications in the toxicity of engineered nanoparticles. Free Radic Biol Med. 2008;44:1689–99. doi:10.1016/j.freeradbiomed.2008.01.028.
75. Song Y, Li X, Du X. Exposure to nanoparticles is related to pleural effusion, pulmonary fibrosis and granuloma. Eur Respir J. 2009;34:559–67. doi:10.1183/09031936.00178308.

76. Hussain S, Vanoirbeek JAJ, Luyts K, De Vooght V, Verbeken E, Thomassen LCJ, et al. Lung exposure to nanoparticles modulates an asthmatic response in a mouse model. Eur Respir J. 2011;37:299–309. doi:10.1183/09031936.00168509.

77. Lanone S, Boczkowski J. Titanium and gold nanoparticles in asthma: the bad and the ugly. Eur Respir J. 2011;37:225–7. doi:10.1183/09031936.00140110.

78. Newman KL, Newman LS. Occupational causes of sarcoidosis. Curr Opin Allergy Clin Immunol. 2012;12:145–50. doi:10.1097/ACI.0b013e3283515173.

79. Xiao X, Zeng X, Zhang X, Ma L, Liu X, Yu H, et al. Effects of Caryota mitis profilin-loaded PLGA nanoparticles in a murine model of allergic asthma. Int J Nanomedicine. 2013;8:4553–62. doi:10.2147/IJN.S51633.

80. Shen L, Higuchi T, Tubbe I, Voltz N, Krummen M, Pektor S, et al. A trifunctional dextran-based nanovaccine targets and activates murine dendritic cells, and induces potent cellular and humoral immune responses *in vivo*. PLoS ONE. 2013;8:e80904. doi:10.1371/journal.pone.0080904.

81. Park M-H, Kim J-H, Jeon J-W, Park J-K, Lee B-J, Suh G-H, et al. Preformulation studies of bee venom for the preparation of bee venom-loaded PLGA particles. Molecules. 2015;20:15072–83. doi:10.3390/molecules200815072.

82. Shahbazi M-A, Fernández TD, Mäkilä EM, Le Guével X, Mayorga C, Kaasalainen MH, et al. Surface chemistry dependent immunostimulative potential of porous silicon nanoplatforms. Biomaterials. 2014;35:9224–35. doi:10.1016/j.biomaterials.2014.07.050.

83. Gustafson K, Jakobsen SS, Lorenzen ND, Thyssen JP, Johansen JD, Bonefeld CM, et al. Metal release and metal allergy after total hip replacement with resurfacing versus conventional hybrid prosthesis. Acta Orthop. 2014;85:348–54. doi:10.3109/17453674.2014.922730.

84. Munger MA, Radwanski P, Hadlock GC, Stoddard G, Shaaban A, Falconer J, et al. In vivo human time-exposure study of orally dosed commercial silver nanoparticles. Nanomedicine. 2014;10:1–9. doi:10.1016/j.nano.2013.06.010.

85. Hesterberg TW, Long CM, Lapin CA, Hamade AK, Valberg PA. Diesel exhaust particulate (DEP) and nanoparticle exposures: what do DEP human clinical studies tell us about potential human health hazards of nanoparticles? Inhal Toxicol. 2010;22:679–94. doi:10.3109/08958371003758823.

86. Toyama T, Matsuda H, Ishida I, Tani M, Kitaba S, Sano S, et al. A case of toxic epidermal necrolysis-like dermatitis evolving from contact dermatitis of the hands associated with exposure to dendrimers. Contact Dermatitis. 2008;59:122–3. doi:10.1111/j.1600-0536.2008.01340.x.

87. Journeay WS, Goldman RH. Occupational handling of nickel nanoparticles: a case report. Am J Ind Med. 2014;57:1073–6. doi:10.1002/ajim.22344.

88. Liao H-Y, Chung Y-T, Lai C-H, Lin M-H, Liou S-H. Sneezing and allergic dermatitis were increased in engineered nanomaterial handling workers. Ind Health. 2014;52:199–215.

89. Romagnani Matucci Rossi. L'asma bronchiale. SEE-Firenze; 2004.

Chapter 4
Allergens in Occupational Allergy: Prevention and Management – Focus on Asthma

Mario Di Gioacchino, Luca Di Giampaolo, Veronica D'Ambrosio, Federica Martino, Sara Cortese, Alessia Gatta, Loredana Della Valle, Anila Farinelli, Rocco Mangifesta, Francesco Cipollone, Qiao Niu, and Claudia Petrarca

Abstract This article reviews the main aspects for the prevention and management of occupational asthma due to allergic sensitization in the workplace. An accurate allergen identification and characterization is the essential aspect of the primary prevention. Both high and low molecular weight molecules (the first acting as complete antigens the second as haptens) can induce asthma. Sensitization is a dose-related phenomenon, therefore the lower the exposure the lower the risk of sensitization. Health surveillance is the key action of the secondary prevention; it aims at the early identification of workers with occupational exposure to asthma-causing agents by means of respiratory questionnaires; preplacement and periodic visits, with spirometry; immunologic tests; and further investigations to confirm diagnosis and then remove the person from further exposure. Asthma management

M. Di Gioacchino (✉)
Immuntotoxicology and Allergy Unit & Occupational Biorepository,
Center of Excellence on Aging and Translational Medicine (CeSI-MeT), "G. D'Annunzio"
University Foundation, Chieti, Italy

Department of Medicine and Science of Aging, G. d'Annunzio University, Chieti, Italy
e-mail: digioacc@unich.it

L. Di Giampaolo
Department of Medical Oral and Biotechnological Science, G. d'Annunzio University,
Chieti, Italy

V. D'Ambrosio • F. Martino
Specialization School of Occupational Medicine, G. d'Annunzio University,
c/o CeSI-Met Via Colle dell'Ara, 66100 Chieti, Italy

S. Cortese
Department of Medicine and Science of Aging, G. d'Annunzio University, Chieti, Italy

A. Gatta • L.D. Valle • A. Farinelli • F. Cipollone
Specialization School of Allergy and Clinical Immunology, G. d'Annunzio University,
Chieti, Italy

© Springer Science+Business Media Singapore 2017
T. Otsuki et al. (eds.), *Allergy and Immunotoxicology in Occupational Health*,
Current Topics in Environmental Health and Preventive Medicine,
DOI 10.1007/978-981-10-0351-6_4

may be identified with the tertiary prevention. In this phase other than the pharmacological treatment, the occupational doctor should remove the worker from the exposure, as the reduction of allergens is a negative prognostic factor for a severe decline of lung function. In any case, workers should be informed on the risk they encounter at work for a better outcome of the preventive measures.

Keywords Occupational asthma • Occupational allergy • Work ability • Removal from the exposure • Decline in pulmonary function

Occupational allergy refers to diseases or conditions caused by exposure to substances in the workplace and in whose pathogenesis allergic mechanisms (both types I and IV) are involved [1]. Asthma, rhinitis, conjunctivitis, and dermatitis are the most common forms. The goal of managing occupational diseases is avoiding the onset of the diseases itself by the primary prevention, to be done after an accurate allergen identification and characterization, secondary prevention whose key action is health surveillance, and, finally, tertiary prevention with the disease management [2]. Asthma is the most severe manifestation of occupational allergy with possible outcome in occupational disability. In this chapter we will address the various steps for the prevention of the allergic occupational asthma.

4.1 Primary Prevention

The difficulties in preventing the onset of asthma and allergy in general in internal medicine are all present in the occupational setting. The allergen identification is the first issue. A careful risk assessment, through the environmental monitoring, provides fundamental information about substances encountered on the job, their concentration, and their sources. Such data could be used to direct the engineering actions to be applied in order to avoid exposure to hazardous substances and to evaluate the effectiveness of measures designed to maintain their concentration

R. Mangifesta
Immunotoxicology and Allergy Unit, CeSI, G. d'Annunzio University Foundation,
Chieti, Italy

Q. Niu
Occupational Health Department, Public Health School, Shanxi Medical University,
Shanxy, Taiyuan 030001, China

C. Petrarca
Immuntotoxicology and Allergy Unit & Occupational Biorepository,
Center of Excellence on Aging and Translational Medicine (CeSI-MeT), "G. D'Annunzio"
University Foundation, Chieti, Italy

below the exposure limits [3]. Assessing exposure entails a scrutiny of who does what, where, and how. However, there are frequently objective difficulties in identifying the agent directly responsible for or most closely associated with the risk of occupational allergy, as in the reported cases of occupational asthma due to allergy to molds contaminating the cooling system of the workplace [4]. In any case, there are few possibilities in completely preventing the onset of allergies to occupational allergens. The main debate was to establish the workability of atopic subject who should work in an environment rich in potential allergens. Should this subject be employed, being atopics at risk of developing allergic diseases, including asthma? Recent data seems to indicate that atopy should be considered insufficient to advise against working in environment with aeroallergens, even to cross-sectional studies have shown that the likelihood of sensitization to large molecules of biological origin [5], such as laboratory animal allergens [6], microbial enzymes, and latex glove protein [7], is increased in atopics. On the other hand, smoking seems to be a greater and more significant determinant risk for sensitization compared to atopy [8]. In particular, smoking, and not atopy, appears to be a risk factor for sensitization to low molecular weight (LMW) chemicals [9]. However, neither the atopy nor smoking is sufficiently predictive to be used in determining the ability of a worker to participate in a job that carries a risk of sensitization [10]. Some studies have reported that the exclusion of atopics might still allow employment of more people who would become sensitized than the number of those whose sensitization had been averted in primary prevention. Therefore, evidence of atopy per se is not adequate justification for refusing employment where there is exposure to respiratory allergens [6]. It must be stressed that prevention of work-related diseases should rest primarily on making the workplace safer for workers rather than by using poorly validated criteria for excluding individuals from employment.

The identification of occupational allergens results mainly from reports of health surveillance. However, there is a need for the identification of occupational allergens in an earlier phase, before the onset of asthma, but no established protocols for an efficient prospective identification of chemical respiratory sensitizers are at present available. Recently some authors [11, 12] suggested the possibility to evaluate the structure–activity relationship (SAR) models as potential methods to prospectively conclude on the sensitization potential of LMW chemicals. However, no single SAR model was sufficiently reliable, but combining two SARs with individual applicability domains of the models provided reliable predictions for one-third of the respiratory sensitizers and nonsensitizers analyzed. The authors stated that a positive predictive value of 96 % and a negative predictive value of 89 % were obtained. In any case for the two-thirds of the chemicals, additional information is required (*in chemico* or in vitro methods) to reach a reliable conclusion.

Allergens can be complete antigens or haptens [13]. The first are high molecular weight (HMW) organic compounds (Table 4.1) and the second LMW chemicals that can stimulate the IgE production as hapten–protein conjugate [14]. The list of such substances (Table 4.2) is continuously increasing.

There are many other substances, such as some metals (aluminum, vanadium), fluxes (colophony, ethylethanolamine), insecticides (organophosphates), diisocyanates

Table 4.1 Natural allergens.
Organic compounds of high
molecular weight

Animal protein
Fur, pelts, urine, serum
Insect – arthropods
Mites, locust, honeybee
Plant protein
Grain, rye flour
Enzymes
Animal, plant, and microbial
Legumes
Coffee beans, soybeans
Seeds
Linseed, cottonseeds
Vegetable gums
Guar gum, acacia gum
Miscellaneous
Latex, tobacco, tea, henna

Table 4.2 Inorganic and
organic chemicals of low
molecular weight, known or
suspected allergens

Anhydrides
Phthalic, trimellitic
Metals
Nickel, chromium
Dyes
Paraphenylenediamine
Diisocyanates
MDI, HDI
Antibiotics
Penicillin, spiramycin
Wood dust
Red cedar, ramin
Miscellaneous
Chloramine-T, piperazine, ethylendiamine, persulfate salts, glutaraldehyde, a-methyldopa, triethylene, etc.)

(TDI, NDI, IDI), and others (methyl methacrylate, NO_2, diesel exhaust particles, SO_2, etc.), in the work environment able to induce asthma by an IgE-independent mechanism [15]. They may involve cell-mediated hypersensitivity or act through direct toxic effect [16, 17]. These chemicals can induce the reactive airway dysfunction syndrome. However, they may affect the immune system, and some of them seem also to favor allergen sensitization. As example, it has been demonstrated that diesel exhaust particle exposure results in accumulation of allergen-specific Th2/Th17 cells in the lungs, potentiating secondary allergen recall responses and promoting the development of allergic asthma [18].

High-level irritant exposure may cause ciliary activity decrease, massive damage of epithelial cells, and tight junction disruption. Injured epithelial cells may activate mucosal inflammation in particular stimulating the recruitment of inflammatory cell, particularly eosinophils [19–21]. The direct effect of pollutants on mast cells induces inflammatory mediator and chemotactic factor release, thereby enhancing mucosal inflammation [19–22]. Some chemicals, in particular diesel exhaust particles, phthalates, and some engineered and anthropogenic nanoparticles, may also favor allergic sensitization [23]. In particular, diesel exhaust particles enhance production of mucosal IgE-secreting cells [20], and some toxic agents, such as lead, chromium, platinum, and palladium (these two last produced by vehicular traffic in the urban environment but also present in many working environments), favor the prevalence of Th2 immune pattern of cytokines [24, 25].

Other factors besides the environmental and occupational toxic pollutants may increase the risk of sensitization to occupational allergens. Some HLA markers were found to be associated with sensitization to allergens as cow dander [26], isocyanates [27], and anhydrides [28]. Genetic susceptibility to environmental exposures may contribute to the onset of occupational diseases in the workplace [29]. For diseases with complex and multifactorial etiology such as occupational asthma, susceptibility studies for selected genetic polymorphisms provide additional insight into the biological mechanisms of disease. However, the value of genetic screening in occupational settings remains limited due to primarily ethical and social concerns.

The attention was also focused on the possible effects of electromagnetic fields (ELMF) in human health [30]. The results of such studies are contrasting as some authors reported that ELMFs favor allergic sensitization to environmental allergens inducing a Th2 cytokine pattern [31], while others found an induction of a Th17 cytokine pattern [32].

Improving the workplace design, implementing alternative processes, changing engineering design (extraction, containment of process, ventilation), and substituting the sensitizer with an alternative chemical, although not always feasible, are measures useful in reducing the risk of occupational exposure. Therefore, efforts have been made to reduce exposure to respiratory sensitizers by instituting occupational hygiene measures such as containment, improved ventilation, and (as a last option) the use of personal protective equipment, as well as worker education to enhance adherence to recommended measures. Examples in which one or more of these measures have been effective include the use of latex-free materials in preventing sensitization to latex [33], encapsulation of enzymes in the detergent industry [34], the use of appropriate respiratory and protective devices and skin covering to reduce the exposure to laboratory animals [35], and worker education to reduce exposure in bakeries [36]. The most effective measures for primary prevention are a combination of intervention in the workplace, use of protective equipment, and worker education to the prevention itself [37]. However, the implementation of preventive measures in the workplace is suboptimal even in occupations with a well-recognized risk of sensitization [38].

A further topic to be addressed is the value of the allergen exposure limits for the prevention of occupational respiratory allergies. The statement of the International Labor Organization, made in 1977, considered the exposure limits "…the concentration in air of a harmful substance which, if the standards are respected, does not generally have harmful effects – including long-term effects on posterity – on the health of workers exposed for 8–10 h a day, 40 h a week; this exposure is considered acceptable by the competent authority which determines the limits, but it is possible that it may not completely guarantee the protection of health of all the workers" [39].

Actually, the exposure limits do not constitute an absolute dividing line between the harmless and the harmful concentrations, but is intended solely as a guide to prevention. In any case the exposure limits for toxic substances are not useful for sensitizing agents. As example, sensitization to glutaraldehyde has been reported in healthcare workers, despite its concentration in the workplace was below the exposure limits [40]. However, also the development of allergic sensitization (and the elicitation of an allergic reaction) is a threshold phenomenon. There are levels of exposure below which sensitization will not be acquired as demonstrated by both relevant human studies of occupational asthma and experimental models [41]. Unfortunately, although there is evidence that the acquisition of sensitization to chemical respiratory allergens is a dose-related phenomenon and that thresholds exist, it is frequently difficult to define accurate numerical values for threshold exposure levels. Therefore, it is difficult to set exposure limits below exposures regarded as "safe" in an absolute sense – although the risk might be very low. Moreover, it is possible that once sensitized, the airborne concentrations at which symptoms could be provoked might be even lower than the concentrations responsible for sensitization in the first instance [39].

As stated by the European Respiratory Society (ERS) task force in the guidelines published in 2012 [42], the following measures are of high impact in controlling work-related exposure to prevent asthma:

- Exposure elimination is the strongest preventive approach to reducing the disease burden of work-related asthma and is the preferred primary prevention approach.
- If elimination is not possible, reduction is the second best option for primary prevention of work-related asthma based on exposure–response relationships.
- There is limited evidence of the effectiveness of respirators in preventing occupational asthma, and other options that are higher in the hierarchy of controls for occupational exposures, notably eliminating or minimizing exposures at the source or in the environment, should be used preferentially.
- Do not use powdered allergen-rich natural rubber latex gloves.
- Minimize skin exposure to asthma-inducing agents.

4.2   Secondary Prevention and Heath Surveillance

Health surveillance is the essence of the secondary prevention (Table 4.3). It can be defined as "the set of medical acts, aimed at protecting the health and safety of workers, in relation to the work environment, occupational risk factors and procedures for carrying out work, and at the formulation of the judgment of the specific working task ability."

Table 4.3 Strategies for secondary prevention

Health surveillance
Replacement visit
Periodic examination
Questionnaires
Biological monitoring (Immunologic and functional tests)
Exposure assessment
Using personal protective equipment
Last line of defense in situations where control at source is clearly impracticable: man-made exposures
Worker education

In the case of occupational asthma, secondary prevention includes early identification of workers with occupational exposure to asthma-causing agents by means of medical surveillance that consists of preplacement and periodic visits; respiratory questionnaires, with spirometry; immunologic tests; and further investigations to confirm diagnosis and then remove workers from further exposure.

Preplacement visit includes clinical, instrumental, and laboratory investigations aimed at assessing the state of health prior to the occupational hazard exposure and to identify any congenital or acquired abnormalities that may represent a clinical condition of increased respiratory susceptibility toward the irritating, sensitizing, and toxic substances, to which workers will be exposed. It has the aim to define the ability of workers for the specific task. In occasion of the periodic medical examinations, the investigations are designed to check, in the light of actual exposure conditions, the onset of any early and reversible changes of the respiratory system, caused by occupational exposures. Trends of symptom prevalence, suggesting sensitization in relation to different categories of employees, workplaces, and tasks, should be investigated. In this way, it is possible to control the frequency of the occupational allergies [42], to evaluate the risk of occupational disease among the different jobs [43], and to identify sensitizing substances [44, 45].

Health surveillance enables the early identification of adverse health effects in individuals; it may supplement environmental monitoring in assessing control and may contribute to the process of hazard and risk assessment; it offers information regarding hazardous substances to which the employees are exposed, the symptoms which may result, the potential long-term risks, and, therefore, the need to report these symptoms to the occupational health service.

The use of questionnaires seems to be useful in detecting subjects with occupational asthma, and such measures have been introduced in some companies for at-risk workers employed in bakeries, working with animals, detergents, diisocyanates, or complex platinum salts or exposed to acid anhydrides. Studies suggest that such programs are beneficial [46, 47], although the benefit is difficult to precisely specify. It has been suggested that the questionnaire component is likely to be less reliable among respondents who believe that their answers might result in job loss [48, 49].

Some occupations have a higher prevalence of asthma than other occupations. Data of each industry should be collected with the aim of identifying worker populations with a high burden of asthma to which disease prevention efforts should be targeted. Anyway, striking differences are evident comparing results obtained from health surveillance schemes in different countries, such as for England (SHIELD), Finland, Chicago (SENSOR), and Quebec [50]. However, only some of those differences are real, due to the variation on the type and size of the industries, working practices, and environmental protection in the workplace. For example, the high prevalence of occupational asthma in Finland due to animal allergens compared to the other countries may be explained by different farming practice. On the other hand, occupational asthma in Finland is compensated and reports are compulsory, whereas, in the other countries, cases are based on voluntary reporting from hospital and physicians who are unlikely to be consulted by self-employed and uninsured farmers [51].

Physicians should also consider gender differences when diagnosing and treating asthma in working adults. In fact, among adults with work-related asthma, males and females differ in terms of workplace exposures, occupations, and industries. In a study on 8239 confirmed work-related asthma cases, a significant gender difference in the distribution of the disease has been shown; in fact 60 % of them were females. Females were more likely to have work-aggravated asthma and less likely to have new-onset asthma. Females with asthma worked in healthcare and social assistance, educational services, retail trade industries, office and administrative support, education training and library and as healthcare and technical practitioners. Asthma was induced prevalently by miscellaneous chemicals, cleaning materials, and indoor air pollutant in females and miscellaneous chemicals, mineral and inorganic dusts, and pyrolysis products in males [52].

Some authors report that work-related asthma exposures are not discussed between workers and their healthcare provider and this communication gap has implications for asthma management [53]. In any phase the employee must be informed on the specific risks of asthma associated with the occupation and in the control measures to be applied.

The ERS task force guidelines (2012) for occupational asthma [46] recommend that in performing the medical screening and surveillance, the following issues should be performed:

- Questionnaire-based identification of all workers at risk of developing work-related asthma.
- A preplacement screening in order to identify workers at higher risk of work-related asthma.
- Detection of sensitization either by specific immunoglobulin E or skin prick test.
- Inform atopic subjects and subjects with preemployment sensitization about their increased risk of work-related asthma.
- In all workers with confirmed occupational rhinitis and/or nonspecific bronchial hyperresponsiveness, periodically administer questionnaire, detect sensitization using standardized skin prick tests or serum-specific immunoglobulin E antibodies, and early refer symptomatic and/or sensitized subjects for specialized medical assessment and assessment of asthma.

- Use risk stratification by diagnostic models to select exposed workers for further medical evaluation.
- Carry out exposure assessment (and all possible related interventions) simultaneously to the medical surveillance.

4.3   Tertiary Prevention and Disease Management

Despite applying primary prevention measures and a proper health surveillance, asthma will affect some workers. Literature reports that the population attributable risk of occupational asthma is between 10 and 25 %, equivalent to an incidence of 250–300 cases per one million people per year [54]. Individual cases need to be carefully investigated and managed. The case management includes the disease monitoring with symptom score, inflammatory and immune biomarkers, and functional parameters (Table 4.4). Among immune biomarkers the usefulness of specific IgE in detecting allergies to organic compounds of HMW is well known. Their useful role has also been reported in allergy to LMW [55]. It has been shown that specific IgE to isocyanates and several other LMW chemicals is more specific than sensitive index of occupational sensitization, and their sensitivity is lower when assayed after cessation of the exposure, with a half-life of 1–2 years [56]. Therefore, specific IgE have a valuable role to play not only in the diagnosis but also in the surveillance of exposed workers, since the persistence of high specific IgE levels may indicate the persistence of exposure [56].

Eosinophil cationic protein (ECP) is a relevant biomarker of eosinophilic inflammation in asthmatic patients [57, 58], and the eosinophilic inflammation is associated with a great decline of FEV1 [59]. However, rather than single determinations, the increase in serum ECP between pre- and post- allergen exposures has a strong correlation with clinical parameters and nonspecific bronchial hyperreactivity [60].

Nonspecific bronchial hyperactivity is indeed an early and sensitive marker of bronchial response to occupational allergens. An increase in nonspecific bronchial hyperreactivity has been found in patients with possible occupational asthma in which the specific bronchial challenge was negative [61].

Table 4.4 Strategies for tertiary prevention

Disease monitoring
Biomarkers, PEF, etc.
Treatment of the disease
Guidelines for asthma treatment
Removal of the exposure
As early as possible
Reduction of the exposure
Less effective then removal
Reporting and the consideration of workers compensation while off work

The optimal management of the occupational asthma and allergies in general is the removal of affected workers from the exposure, which in practice may be difficult to achieve. It includes avoidance of certain tasks and exposures and relocation to other areas or processes within the workplace. Recent papers in literature compared the effectiveness of complete removal from exposure to the causative agent with reduction of exposure and continued exposure in the management of occupational asthma. Results suggested that complete removal from exposure resulted in the best outcome in terms of symptoms, lung function, and airway hyperresponsiveness. Reduction of exposure appeared to be less effective in terms of improving asthma but was also less likely to result in loss of income or unemployment [62]. Some authors reported that a reduction of exposure was associated with a lower likelihood of improvement and recovery of asthma symptoms and a higher risk of worsening of the symptoms and nonspecific bronchial hyperresponsiveness, compared with complete avoidance of exposure [63]. The decline in pulmonary function in asthmatic workers is particularly severe in those unable to avoid allergen exposure. In fact, it has been reported that, despite an optimal pharmacological therapy, the pulmonary function decay slope was steeper in workers continuously exposed to the sensitizing agent (even at reduced level) than in those with a complete cessation of exposure: final FEV1 loss was 512.5 ± 180 ml versus 332.5 ± 108 ml, respectively. The difference became significant after 4 years from the cessation of the exposure. The study shows that the cessation of the exposure to allergen in the workplace appears the most effective measure in limiting pulmonary function decline in asthmatic workers and underlines the importance of allergic risk assessment and control in the management of occupational asthma [64].

Critical analysis of available evidence indicates the following: 1) persistent exposure to the causal agent is more likely to result in asthma worsening than complete avoidance; (2) there is insufficient evidence to determine whether pharmacological treatment can alter the course of asthma in subjects who remain exposed; (3) avoidance of exposure leads to recovery of asthma in less than one-third of affected workers; (4) reduction of exposure seems to be less beneficial than complete avoidance of exposure; and (5) personal respiratory equipment does not provide complete protection [65].

In some cases the causative allergen-inducing asthma is present also outside the workplace and this situation represents a negative prognostic factor. This is the case of latex that affects a large population of healthcare workers [66, 67]. In the occupational setting, latex gloves and other latex-made equipment have been replaced with powder-free latex or nitrile gloves of latex-free compounds with a reduction of latex-induced diseases including asthma [33]. However, although there was improvement after implementation of powder-free latex gloves, there are still a considerable number of healthcare workers with latex-related asthma symptoms, likely due to nonoccupational latex exposure [68].

Recommendations made by the ERS task force on the management of work-related asthma [42] suggest that:

- Patients, physicians, and employers should be informed that persistence of exposure to the causal agent is likely to result in a deterioration of asthma symptoms and airway obstruction.
- Patients and their attending physicians should be aware that complete avoidance of exposure is associated with the highest probability of improvement, but may not lead to a complete recovery from asthma.
- Reduction of exposure to the causal agent can be considered an alternative to complete avoidance, but this approach requires careful medical monitoring in order to ensure an early identification of asthma worsening.
- The use of respiratory protective equipment should not be regarded as a safe approach, especially in the long term and in patients with severe asthma.
- Anti-asthma medications should not be regarded as a reasonable alternative to environmental interventions.

A further possibility to treat occupational asthma has recently been introduced with the specific immunotherapy that has been tested for a few occupational sensitizing agents with IgE-dependent reactions [69], in particular healthcare workers who were allergic to latex [70] but also in small number of workers who were allergic to cereal [71], sea squirt (Hoya asthma) [72], and laboratory animals [73]. The authors reported encouraging results, but whether asthma outcomes are altered in the long term remains to be determined, and further studies are needed before immunotherapy can be recommended.

Also the use of anti-IgE has shown promising results particularly in severe asthmatic workers. During treatment, nine of the ten treated patients exhibited a lower rate of asthma exacerbations and used less oral or inhaled corticosteroids. Seven patients were able to continue working at the same workplace as before treatment [74]. However, as for the immunotherapy, also anti-IgE requires further prospective studies to be introduced as routine treatment in occupational asthma.

The last resort of the tertiary prevention is the removal of the patient entirely from the workplace. Unfortunately, removal from the exposure is not always associated with a complete recovery from the disease [75, 76]. Table 4.5 reports the negative prognostic factor for the persistence of bronchial obstruction after the removal from the exposure [77–79].

Table 4.5 Negative prognostic factor for the persistence of bronchial obstruction after the removal from the exposure in workers affected by occupational asthma

Type of causal allergen, in particular LMW substances (such as diisocyanates, colophony fumes, and platinum salts)
Long duration of symptoms before diagnosis
Severity of symptoms and airway obstruction at the time of cessation of exposure
Dual response after specific challenge test
Persistence of markers of inflammation in BAL and in induced sputum
Prior history of wheezing or of smoking

Employees suffering from an occupational asthma are often retired or dismissed on "medical grounds." The society should assist the patient with a workers' compensation claim when applicable, to limit the socioeconomic effects of the diagnosis.

In this case, two specific questions need to be answered with regard to such a decision on grounds of occupational asthma:

– Is the employee not well enough in terms of physical capacity to perform work, and so likely to remain unwell that no other job is possible for that particular employee?
– Second, are all the possible jobs so unsafe, because of exposure to the sensitizer or to nonspecific irritants, that this employee could not undertake any such jobs without significant risks to his health and safety?

Of course all efforts for therapeutic management of the suffering worker are to be pursued in any case.

References

1. Peden D, Reed CE. Environmental and occupational allergies. J Allergy Clin Immunol. 2010;125 Suppl 2:S150–60. doi:10.1016/j.jaci.2009.10.073.
2. Tarlo SM, Lemiere C. Occupational asthma. N Engl J Med. 2014;370(7):640–9. doi:10.1056/NEJMra1301758.
3. Nicholson PJ, Cullinan P, Newman Taylor AJ, Burge PS, Boyle C. Evidence based guidelines for the prevention, identification, and management of occupational asthma. Occup Environ Med. 2005;62:290–9.
4. Boscolo P, Piccolomini R, Benvenuti F, Catamo G, Di Gioacchino M. Sensitisation to aspergillus fumigatus and penicillium notatum in laboratory workers. Int J Immunopathol Pharmacol. 1999;12:43–8.
5. Vandenplas O. Occupational asthma: etiologies and risk factors. Allergy Asthma Immunol Res. 2011;3:157–67. doi:10.4168/aair.2011.3.3.157.
6. Krop EJ, Heederik DJ, Lutter R, de Meer G, Aalberse RC, Jansen HM, et al. Associations between pre-employment immunologic and airway mucosal factors and the development of occupational allergy. J Allergy Clin Immunol. 2009;123:694–700. doi:10.1016/j.jaci.2008.12.021.
7. Bernstein DI, Malo JL. High molecular weight agents. In: Bernstein IL, editor. Asthma in the workplace. New York: Marcel Dekker; 1993.
8. Adisesh A, Gruszka L, Robinson E, Evans G. Smoking status and immunoglobulin E seropositivity to workplace allergens. Occup Med (London). 2011;61:62–4.
9. Venables KM. Low molecular weight chemicals hypersensitivity and direct toxicity: the acid anhydrides. Br J Ind Med. 1989;46:222–32.
10. Wilken D, Baur X, Barbinova L, Preisser A, Meijer E, Rooyackers J, et al. What are the benefits of medical screening and surveillance? Eur Respir Rev. 2012;21:105–11.
11. Dik S, Ezendam J, Cunningham AR, Carrasquer CA, van Loveren H, Rorije E. Evaluation of *in silico* models for the identification of respiratory sensitizers. Toxicol Sci. 2014;142:385–94. doi:10.1093/toxsci/kfu188.
12. Seed MJ, Cullinan P, Agius RM. Methods for the prediction of low-molecular-weight occupational respiratory sensitizers. Curr Opin Allergy Clin Immunol. 2008;8:103–9. doi:10.1097/ACI.0b013e3282f4cadd.

13. Malo JL, Chan-Yeung M. Agents causing occupational asthma. J Allergy Clin Immunol. 2009;123:545–50.
14. Isola D, Kimber I, Sarlo K, Lalko J, Sipes IG. Chemical respiratory allergy and occupational asthma: what are the key areas of uncertainty? J Appl Toxicol. 2008;28:249–53.
15. Kimber I, Agius R, Basketter DA, Corsini E, Cullinan P, Dearman RJ, et al. Chemical respiratory allergy: opportunities for hazard identification and characterization: the report and recommendations of ECVAM Workshop 60. Altern Lab Anim. 2007;35:243–65.
16. Wantke F, Focke M, Hemmer W, Bracun R, Wolf-Abdolvahab S, Götz M, et al. Exposure to formaldehyde and phenol during an anatomy dissecting course: sensitizing potency of formaldehyde in medical students. Allergy. 2000;55:84–7.
17. Bernstein DI, Bernstein IL. Occupational asthma. In: Middleton E, Reed CE, Ellis EF, Adkinson NF, Yunginger JW, Busse WW, editors. Allergy: principles & practice. St. Louis: Mosby; 1998. p. 963–80.
18. Brandt EB, Biagini Myers JM, Acciani TH, Ryan PH, Sivaprasad U, Ruff B, et al. Exposure to allergen and diesel exhaust particles potentiates secondary allergen-specific memory responses, promoting asthma susceptibility. J Allergy Clin Immunol. 2015;136:295–303. doi:10.1016/j.jaci.2014.11.043.
19. Norback D, Wålinder R, Wieslander G, Smedje G, Erwall C, Venge P. Indoor air pollutants in schools: nasal and biomarkers in nasal lavage. Allergy. 2000;55:163–70.
20. Riedl MA, Diaz-Sanchez D, Linn WS, Gong Jr H, Clark KW, Effros RM, et al. Allergic inflammation in the human lower respiratory tract affected by exposure to diesel exhaust. Res Rep Health Eff Inst. 2012;165:5–43.
21. Ciencewicki J, Trivedi S, Kleeberger SR. Oxidants and the pathogenesis of lung diseases. J Allergy Clin Immunol. 2008;122:456–68.
22. Kunkel G, Schierhorn K. Air pollution and allergic and non-allergic airway disease. ACI Int. 1999;11:82–5.
23. Lefebvre DE, Pearce B, Fine JH, Chomyshyn E, Ross N, Halappanavar S, et al. In vitro enhancement of mouse T helper 2 cell sensitization to ovalbumin allergen by carbon black nanoparticles. Toxicol Sci. 2014;138:322–32. doi:10.1093/toxsci/kfu010.
24. Boscolo P, Di Gioacchino M, Sabbioni E, Di Giacomo F, Reale M, Volpe AR, et al. Lymphocyte subpopulations, cytokine and trace elements in asymptomatic atopic women exposed to an urban environment. Life Sci. 2000;67:1119–26.
25. Di Gioacchino M, Verna N, Di Giampaolo L, Di Claudio F, Turi MC, Perrone A, et al. Immunotoxicity and sensitizing capacity of metal compounds depend on speciation. Int J Immunopathol Pharmacol. 2007;20(2 Suppl 2):15–22.
26. Kauppinen A, Peräsaari J, Taivainen A, Kinnunen T, Saarelainen S, Rytkönen-Nissinen M, et al. Association of HLA class II alleles with sensitization to cow dander Bos d 2, an important occupational allergen. Immunobiology. 2012;217:8–12. doi:10.1016/j.imbio.2011.08.012.
27. Palikhe NS, Kim JH, Park HS. Biomarkers predicting isocyanate-induced asthma. Allergy Asthma Immunol Res. 2011;3:21–6. doi:10.4168/aair.2011.3.1.21.
28. Young RP, Barker RD, Pile KD, Cookson WO, Taylor AJ. The association of HLA-DR3 with specific IgE to inhaled acid anhydrides. Am J Respir Crit Care Med. 1995;151:219–21.
29. Christiani DC, Mehta AJ, Yu CL. Genetic susceptibility to occupational exposures. Occup Environ Med. 2008;65:430–6. doi:10.1136/oem.2007.033977.
30. Cossarizza A, Monti D, Bersani F, Paganelli R, Montagnani G, Cadossi R, et al. Extremely low frequency pulsed electromagnetic fields increase interleukin-2 (IL2) utilization and IL-2 receptor expression in mitogen-stimulated human lymphocytes from old subjects. FEBS Lett. 1989;8:141–4.
31. Boscolo P, Di Sciascio MB, Benvenuti F, Reale M, Di Stefano F, Conti P, et al. Effects of low frequency electromagnetic fields on expression of lymphocyte subsets and production of cytokines of men and women employed in a museum. Sci Total Environ. 2001;270:13–20.

32. Salehi I, Sani KG, Zamani A. Exposure of rats to extremely low-frequency electromagnetic fields (ELF-EMF) alters cytokines production. Electromagn Biol Med. 2013;32:1–8. doi:10.3 109/15368378.2012.692343.
33. Latza U, Haamann F, Baur X. Effectiveness of a nationwide interdisciplinary preventive programme for latex allergy. Int Arch Occup Environ Health. 2005;78:394–402.
34. Sarlo K. Control of occupational asthma and allergy in the detergent industry. Ann Allergy Asthma Immunol. 2003;90 Suppl 2:32–4.
35. Gordon S, Preece R. Prevention of laboratory animal allergy. Occup Med (Lond). 2003;53:371–7.
36. Fishwick D, Harris-Roberts J, Robinson E, Evans G, Barraclough R, Sen D, et al. Impact of worker education on respiratory symptoms and sensitization in bakeries. Occup Med (Lond). 2011;61:321–7.
37. Ghittori S, Ferrari M, Negri S, Serranti P, Sacco P, Biffi R, et al. Recent prevention strategies and occupational risk analysis: control Banding and Sobane. G Ital Med Lav Ergon. 2006;28:30–43.
38. Stave GM, Darcey DJ. Prevention of laboratory animal allergy in the United States: a national survey. J Occup Environ Med. 2012;54:558–63.
39. Hunter WJ, Aresini G, Haigh R, Papadopoulos P, Von der Hude W. Occupational exposure limits for chemicals in the European Union. Occup Environ Med. 1997;54:217–22.
40. Di Stefano F, Siriruttanapruk S, McCoach J, Burge PS. Glutaraldehyde: an occupational hazard in the hospital setting. Allergy. 1999;54:1105–9.
41. Cochrane SA, Arts JH, Ehnes C, Hindle S, Hollnagel HM, Poole A, et al. Thresholds in chemical respiratory sensitisation. Toxicology. 2015;333:179–94. doi:10.1016/j.tox.2015.04.010.
42. Baur X, Sigsgaard T, Aasen TB, Burge PS, Heederik D, Henneberger P, et al. Guidelines for the management of work-related asthma. Eur Respir J. 2012;39:529–45. doi:10.1183/09031936.00096111.
43. Kogevinas M, Antó JM, Sunyer J, Tobias A, Kromhout H, Burney P. Occupational asthma in Europe and other industrialized areas: a population-based study. Lancet. 1999;353:1750–4.
44. Di Stefano F, Verna N, Di Giampaolo L, Schiavone C, Di Gioacchino G, Balatsinou L, et al. Occupational asthma due to low molecular weight agents. Int J Immunopathol Pharmacol. 2004;17(2 Suppl):77–82.
45. Di Stefano F, Siriruttanapruk S, McCoach J, Di Gioacchino M, Burge PS. Occupational asthma in a highly industrialized region of UK: report from a local surveillance scheme. Eur Ann Allergy Clin Immunol. 2004;36:56–62.
46. Buyantseva LV, Liss GM, Ribeiro M, Manno M, Luce CE, Tarlo SM. Reduction in diisocyanate and non-diisocyanate sensitizer-induced occupational asthma in Ontario. J Occup Environ Med. 2011;53:420–6.
47. Allan KM, Murphy E, Ayres JG. Assessment of respiratory health surveillance for laboratory animal workers. Occup Med (Lond). 2010;60:458–63.
48. Suarthana E, Vergouwe Y, Moons KG, de Monchy J, Grobbee D, Heederik D, et al. A diagnostic model for the detection of sensitization to wheat allergens was developed and validated in bakery workers. J Clin Epidemiol. 2010;63:1011–9.
49. Meijer E, Suarthana E, Rooijackers J, Grobbee DE, Jacobs JH, Meijster T, et al. Application of a prediction model for work-related sensitisation in bakery workers. Eur Respir J. 2010;36:735–42.
50. Meredith S, Nordman H. Occupational asthma: measures of frequency form four countries. Torax. 1996;51:453–40.
51. Tarlo SM, Liss G, Corey P, Broder I. A workers compensation claim population for occupational asthma. Comparison of subgroups. Chest. 1995;107:634–41.
52. White GE, Seaman C, Filios MS, Mazurek JM, Flattery J, Harrison RJ, et al. Gender differences in work-related asthma: surveillance data from California, Massachusetts, Michigan, and New Jersey, 1993–2008. J Asthma. 2014;51:691–702. doi:10.3109/02770903.2014.90396 8.

53. Anderson NJ, Fan ZJ, Reeb-Whitaker C, Bonauto DK, Rauser E. Distribution of asthma by occupation: Washington State behavioral risk factor surveillance system data, 2006–2009. J Asthma. 2014;51:1035–42. doi:10.3109/02770903.2014.939282.

54. Kogevinas M, Zock JP, Jarvis D, Kromhout H, Lillienberg L, Plana E, Radon K, et al. Exposure to substances in the work- place and new-onset asthma: an international prospective population-based study (ECRHS-II). Lancet. 2007;370:336–41.

55. Blindow S, Preisser AM, Baur X, Budnik LT. Is the analysis of histamine and/or interleukin-4 release after isocyanate challenge useful in the identification of patients with IgE-mediated isocyanate asthma? J Immunol Methods. 2015;422:35–50. doi:10.1016/j.jim.2015.03.024.

56. Tee RD, Cullinan P, Welch J, Burge PS, Newman-Taylor AJ. Specific IE to isocyanate: a useful diagnostic role in occupational asthma. J Allergy Clin Immunol. 1998;101:709–15.

57. Koh GC, Shek LP, Goh DY, Van Bever H, Koh DS. Eosinophil cationic protein: is it useful in asthma? A systematic review. Respir Med. 2007;101:696–705.

58. Venge P. The eosinophil and airway remodelling in asthma. Clin Respir J. 2010;4 Suppl 1:15–9. doi:10.1111/j.1752-699X.2010.00192.x.

59. Talini D, Novelli F, Bacci E, Bartoli M, Cianchetti S, Costa F, et al. Sputum eosinophilia is a determinant of FEV1 decline in occupational asthma: results of an observational study. BMJ Open. 2015;5:e005748. doi:10.1136/bmjopen-2014-005748.

60. Di Gioacchino M, Cavallucci E, Di Stefano F, Verna N, Ramondo S, Ciuffreda S, et al. Influence of total IgE and seasonal increase of eosinophil cationic protein on bronchial hyper-reactivity in asthmatic grass-sensitized farmers. Allergy. 2000;55:1030–4.

61. Jares EJ, Baena-Cagnani CE, Gómez RM. Diagnosis of occupational asthma: an update. Curr Allergy Asthma Rep. 2012;12:221–31. doi:10.1007/s11882-012-0259-2.

62. Birdi K, Beach J. Management of sensitizer-induced occupational asthma: avoidance or reduction of exposure? Curr Opin Allergy Clin Immunol. 2013;13:132–7. doi:10.1097/ACI.0b013e32835ea249.

63. Vandenplas O, Dressel H, Wilken D, Jamart J, Heederik D, Maestrelli P, et al. Management of occupational asthma: cessation or reduction of exposure? A systematic review of available evidence. Eur Respir J. 2011;38:804–11. doi:10.1183/09031936.00177510.

64. Di Giampaolo L, Cavallucci E, Braga M, Renzetti A, Schiavone C, Quecchia C, et al. The persistence of allergen exposure favors pulmonary function decline in workers with allergic occupational asthma. Int Arch Occup Environ Health. 2012;85:181–8. doi:10.1007/s00420-011-0653-4.

65. Vandenplas O, Dressel H, Nowak D, Jamart J, ERS Task Force on the Management of Work-related Asthma. What is the optimal management option for occupational asthma? Eur Respir Rev. 2012;21:97–104. doi:10.1183/09059180.00004911.

66. Walters GI, Moore VC, McGrath EE, Burge PS, Henneberger PK. Agents and trends in health care workers' occupational asthma. Occup Med (Lond). 2013;63:513–6. doi:10.1093/occmed/kqt093.

67. Verna N, Di Giampaolo L, Renzetti A, Balatsinou L, Di Stefano F, Di Gioacchino G, et al. Prevalence and risk factors for latex-related diseases among healthcare workers in an Italian general hospital. Ann Clin Lab Sci. 2003;33:184–91.

68. Nienhaus A, Kromark K, Raulf-Heimsoth M, van Kampen V, Merget R. Outcome of occupational latex allergy – work ability and quality of life. PLoS One. 2008;3:e3459. doi:10.1371/journal.pone.0003459.

69. Crivellaro M, Senna G, Marcer G, Passalacqua G. Immunological treatments for occupational allergy. Int J Immunopathol Pharmacol. 2013;26:579–84.

70. Moscato G, Pala G, Sastre J. Specific immunotherapy and biological treatments for occupational allergy. Curr Opin Allergy Clin Immunol. 2014;14:576–81. doi:10.1097/ACI.0000000000000105.

71. Armentia A, Martin-Santos JM, Quintero A, Fernandez A, Barber D, Alonso E, et al. Bakers' asthma: prevalence and evaluation of immunotherapy with a wheat flour extract. Ann Allergy. 1990;65:265–72.

72. Jyo T, Kodomari Y, Kodomari N, Kuwabara W, Katsutani T, Otsuka T, et al. Therapeutic effect and titers of the specific IgE and IgG antibodies in patients with sea squirt allergy (Hoya asthma) un- der a long-term hyposensitization with three sea squirt antigens. J Allergy Clin Immunol. 1989;83:386–93.

73. Hansen I, Hörmann K, Klimek L. Specific immunotherapy in inhalative allergy to rat epithelium. Laryngorhinootologie. 2004;83:512–5 (in German).

74. Lavaud F, Bonniaud P, Dalphin JC, Leroyer C, Muller D, Tannous R, et al. Usefulness of omalizumab in ten patients with severe occupational asthma. Allergy. 2013;68:813–5. doi:10.1111/all.12149.

75. Labrecque M, Khemici E, Cartier A, Malo JL, Turcot J. Impairment in workers with isocyanate-induced occupational asthma and removed from exposure in the province of Québec between 1985 and 2002. J Occup Environ Med. 2006;48:1093–8.

76. Rüegger M, Droste D, Hofmann M, Jost M, Miedinger D. Diisocyanate-induced asthma in Switzerland: long-term course and patients' self-assessment after a 12-year follow-up. J Occup Med Toxicol. 2014;9:21. doi:10.1186/1745-6673-9-21.

77. Broding HC, Frank P, Hoffmeyer F, Bünger J. Course of occupational asthma depending on the duration of workplace exposure to allergens – a retrospective cohort study in bakers and farmers. Ann Agric Environ Med. 2011;18:35–40.

78. Descatha A, Leproust H, Choudat D, Garnier R, Pairon JC, Ameille J. Factors associated with severity of occupational asthma with a latency period at diagnosis. Allergy. 2007;62:795–801.

79. Maestrelli P, Schlünssen V, Mason P, Sigsgaard T, ERS Task Force on the Management of Work-related Asthma. Contribution of host factors and workplace exposure to the outcome of occupational asthma. Eur Respir Rev. 2012;21:88–96. doi:10.1183/09059180.00004811.

Chapter 5
Particulate-Driven Type-2 Immunity and Allergic Responses

Etsushi Kuroda, Burcu Temizoz, Cevayir Coban, Koji Ozasa, and Ken J. Ishii

Abstract It is thought that particle pollutants exacerbate allergic responses that are defined as highly increased airway cellular responses and IgE production. These particulates are nanometer- to micrometer-sized particles such as particulate matter 2.5 (PM2.5), diesel exhaust particles, and Asian sand dust (ASD). Other than particle pollutants, particulates with similar sizes such as aluminum salts (alum) and silica are also known to induce type-2 immune responses that are characterized by the activation of eosinophils and the induction of antigen-specific serum IgE in vivo. All of these particulates have a common feature in that they function as adjuvants and promote antigen-specific immune responses. An adjuvant is an activator of innate immunity, and innate immunity is thought to be required for the adequate induction of adaptive immunity. In general, innate immune cells are activated through pattern recognition receptors (PRRs) such as Toll-like receptors (TLRs) and

E. Kuroda (✉) • K.J. Ishii (✉)
Laboratory of Vaccine Science, WPI Immunology Frontier Research Center (IFReC),
Osaka University, 3-1 Yamada-oka, Suita, Osaka 565-0871, Japan

Laboratory of Vaccine Design, Center for Drug Design Research, National Institute
of Biomedical Innovation, Health and Nutrition (NIBIOHN), Osaka, Japan

Laboratory of Adjuvant Innovation, National Institute of Biomedical Innovation,
Health and Nutrition (NIBIOHN), Osaka, Japan
e-mail: kuroetu@ifrec.osaka-u.ac.jp; kenishii@biken.osaka-u.ac.jp

B. Temizoz
Laboratory of Vaccine Science, WPI Immunology Frontier Research Center (IFReC),
Osaka University, 3-1 Yamada-oka, Suita, Osaka 565-0871, Japan

C. Coban
Laboratory of Malaria Immunology, WPI Immunology Frontier Research Center (IFReC),
Osaka University, 3-1 Yamada-oka, Suita, Osaka 565-0871, Japan

K. Ozasa
Laboratory of Adjuvant Innovation, National Institute of Biomedical Innovation,
Health and Nutrition (NIBIOHN), Osaka 567-0085, Japan

Department of Pediatrics, Yokohama City University Graduate School of Medicine,
Yokohama, Kanagawa 236-0004, Japan

© Springer Science+Business Media Singapore 2017
T. Otsuki et al. (eds.), *Allergy and Immunotoxicology in Occupational Health*,
Current Topics in Environmental Health and Preventive Medicine,
DOI 10.1007/978-981-10-0351-6_5

induce inflammatory responses. However, the basis for the adjuvanticity of these particulates including particle pollutants and the mechanisms by which they elicit allergic responses are still unclear. In addition, not all particulate adjuvants induce allergic responses. In this review, we will discuss the proposed mechanisms behind the activity of particulate adjuvants and their role in exacerbation of allergic inflammation.

Keywords Particulates • Adjuvants • Type-2 immunity • IgE • Damage-associated molecular patterns • Innate immunity

Abbreviations

ASC	Apoptosis-associated speck-like protein containing a caspase recruitment domain
ASD	Asian sand dust
CGAMP	Cyclic GMP-AMP
CGAS	Cyclic GMP-AMP synthase
CLR	C-type lectin receptor
CNT	Carbon nanotube
DAMP	Damage-associated molecular pattern
DC	Dendritic cell
DEP	Diesel exhaust particle
GC	Germinal center
ILC2	Group 2 innate lymphoid cell
IRF	Interferon regulatory factor
KO	Knockout
MSU	Monosodium urate
NKT cell	Natural killer T cell
OVA	Ovalbumin
PAMP	Pathogen-associated molecular pattern
PG	Prostaglandin
PGLA	Poly(lactide-co-glycolide)
PM2.5	Particulate matter 2.5
PRR	Pattern recognition receptor
PTGS	PGE synthase
STAT	Signal transducer and activator of transcription
STING	Stimulator of interferon genes
Syk	Spleen tyrosine kinase
TBK	TANK-binding kinase
Tfh cell	Follicular helper T cell
TLR	Toll-like receptor
WT	Wild type

5.1 Introduction

Recently, the number of patients suffering from allergic disease such as asthma or rhinitis has increased especially in developed countries. The reason for this increase remains unclear, but many studies have demonstrated that particle pollutants such as diesel exhaust particles (DEPs) and ASD may be involved in the exacerbation of allergic responses [1–8]. In fact, epidemiological studies have reported that increased particulate matter in air was significantly associated with increased asthma hospitalization [9, 10]. Allergic responses are mediated by type-2 immune responses, characterized by activation of eosinophils and induction of antigen-specific serum IgE in vivo [11]. Some particulates and crystals, including particle pollutants, are known to stimulate immune responses to induce and enhance type-2 immune responses [12–17]. These particulates are thought to function as adjuvants; for example, alum is a recognized and widely used particulate adjuvant [18–20]. Alum has been used as a human vaccine adjuvant for more than 80 years; however, the detailed mechanism of action of alum is yet to be determined. Thus, the basis for the adjuvanticity of these particulates including particle pollutants and the mechanisms by which they elicit allergic responses remain poorly understood.

5.2 Innate Immunity and Adaptive Immunity

Immune responses are categorized into two types: innate and adaptive [21, 22]. Macrophage and dendritic cells (DCs) are major players in innate immunity. They engulf pathogens or antigens as the first line of defense and then transmit information to the adaptive immune systems via antigen presentation. Adaptive immunity is mediated by T cells, B cells, and memory cells, which all contribute to antigen-specific immune responses. Interestingly, recent studies have demonstrated that innate immunity is required for the adequate induction of adaptive immunity [21–23]. In general, innate immune cells are activated by pathogens or pathogen-derived factors (e.g., pathogen-associated molecular patterns or PAMPs) through PRRs, such as TLRs. Then PRRs transduce activating signals into cells and induce adaptive immunity (Fig. 5.1) [24–27]. In addition to PAMPs, factors released by cell death (damage-associated molecular patterns or DAMPs) also activate PRRs on innate cells to induce inflammatory responses. Lipids, sugars, metabolites, nucleic acids, and cytokines are all categorized as DAMPs, and activation of innate immunity by DAMPs is considered to be critical for adjuvant activity [28–36]. Thus, both exogenous and endogenous factors act as adjuvants activating innate immune cells and inducing adaptive responses.

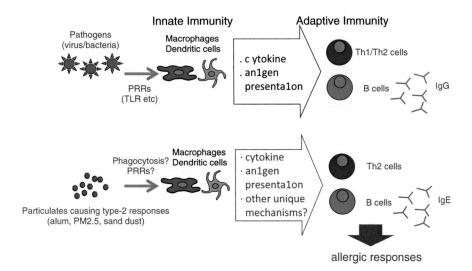

Fig. 5.1 Innate immunity is required for the induction of adaptive immunity. Innate cells sense pathogen via PRRs such as TLR, and then PRRs transduce activating signals into cells. Activated innate cells induce inflammatory responses and promote the activation of adaptive immunity. However, mechanism of action of particulate adjuvant remains poorly understood

5.3   Particulate-Induced Immune Responses

Many studies have reported the adjuvant activity of particulate matter and particulate-induced allergic inflammation [1–8, 12–17]. Representative examples of immune responses induced by particulate matter are presented below.

5.3.1   Particle Pollutants

The most well-known particle pollutant is DEPs. In a mouse model, DEPs functioned as adjuvant and induced ovalbumin (OVA)-specific IgE responses, infiltration of eosinophils, and goblet cell hyperplasia [5, 7]. Similar to DEP, ASD, an aerosol from central and northwestern China that is considered to affect respiratory health, has also been reported to induce allergic inflammation in the lung. Like DEPs, ASD is thought to function as an adjuvant inducing allergen (OVA)-specific responses [3, 4]. A recent study demonstrated that particulate matter 2.5 (PM2.5 is defined as having a particulate size of around or less than 2.5 μm in diameter), present in air, exacerbated allergic lung inflammation in OVA-sensitized and challenged asthmatic mice [37]. In addition, another study showed that intranasal administration of PM2.5 exacerbated allergic lung inflammation in allergy-prone NC/Nga mice [38]. These results suggested that PM2.5 may increase the risk of allergic asthma in allergy-prone children.

5.3.2 Inorganic Particles

Many studies have shown that metal-, chemical-, and mineral-derived particulates have strong adjuvant activity. The most well-known inorganic particulate for immunologists is alum. In general, alum adjuvant preferentially activates humoral immunity to induce antigen-specific antibody responses [18–20]. However, alum is frequently used to generate mouse models of allergic diseases because it strongly induces type-2 immune responses. Similar to alum, crystalline silica is also reported to induce antigen-specific IgE and IgG1 in a mouse model [15]. A recent study demonstrated that inorganic crystalline materials consisting of heterogeneous layers of double hydroxides, such as lithium aluminum, calcium aluminum, and magnesium aluminum, have strong adjuvant activities and induce high levels of antigen-specific IgE [39]. Nickel is a representative allergen that induces contact dermatitis, and nickel oxide nanoparticles also function as type-2 immune adjuvants inducing IgE [14].

5.3.3 Biological Particulates and Metabolites

Several particulates and crystals are generated in the body and induce immune responses through their adjuvanticity. Monosodium urate (MSU) crystals are generated from saturating concentration of uric acid and are the causative agent of gout. Since uric acid is released from damaged cells, MSU crystals are thought to be DAMPs and exhibit strong type-2 adjuvant activity [12, 34, 40–42]. Recent studies demonstrated that MSU crystals play a pivotal role in house dust mite antigen-induced allergic lung inflammation [43]. Chitin is a component of the cell wall of fungi, helminth, and insects. Chitin particles, which are biopolymers of N-acetyl-D-glucosamine, can elicit type-2 immune responses through the induction of interleukin (IL)-4 from eosinophils and basophils [17].

5.3.4 Artificial Particulates

Carbon nanotubes (CNTs) are a well-known carbon nanomaterial with a cylindrical structure that have been applied for use in drug delivery and as semiconductors. Several studies have indicated that CNTs induce lung inflammation [44, 45]. In addition, recent studies have demonstrated that subcutaneous, intranasal, or intratracheal instillation of CNTs plus OVA significantly induced OVA-specific IgE in serum and infiltration of eosinophils in the lung. As with other particulates, CNTs function as type-2 adjuvants to induce antigen-specific Th2 responses [6, 8]. It is not only cylindrical carbon structures that display adjuvant activity; carbon black, a colloidal carbon particle, also possesses adjuvant activity and particularly in ultra-fine form enhanced antigen-specific IgE and induced allergic airway inflammation [46–48].

5.3.5 Particulate Adjuvant Not Causing Allergic Inflammation

Induction of type-2 responses is one of the features of particulate adjuvant; however not all particulates induce allergic inflammation. The biocrystalline substance hemozoin is a hemin detoxification by-product of malaria parasites. Hemozoin and synthetic hemozoin (also known as β-hematin) that do not induce allergic inflammation display strong adjuvant activity [49, 50]. Recently, synthetic hemozoin was tested as a potential influenza vaccine adjuvant [51, 52]. Poly(lactide-co-glycolide) (PGLA) is a biodegradable polymeric nanoparticle that initially attracted attention as a potent delivery system [53]. However, this particle also displays adjuvant activity inducing antigen-specific IgG1 and IgG2c [53, 54]. Interestingly, PGLA stimulates innate cells such as DCs to produce IL-1α and IL-1β through PRR activation [54]. Recently, we reported that hydroxyapatite nanoparticles function as a vaccine adjuvant [55]. The hydroxyapatite particle is a less-toxic particulate adjuvant due to its characteristic of biodegradation and is a promising influenza vaccine adjuvant, similar to PGLA.

Thus, not all but most of the particulates described above function as adjuvants to enhance antigen (allergen)-specific type-2 immune responses. Therefore, it has been hypothesized that particulate adjuvants causing allergy evoke similar and unique signals in innate cells to preferentially activate type-2 immune responses.

5.4 Molecular Mechanisms of Action of Particulate Adjuvants Causing Type-2 Immunity

Many scientists have investigated the mechanisms of action of particulate adjuvants; however, detailed elucidation is yet to be reported. Many potential mechanisms have been proposed, particularly focusing on the activation of innate immune responses by particulate adjuvants. The findings of these studies are detailed below.

5.4.1 TLR and MyD88 Signaling

TLR and MyD88 signaling is one of the major signaling pathways for the activation of innate cells such as macrophages and DCs. Schnare et al. investigated the effect of the particulate adjuvant alum on IgG and IgE responses in MyD88-deficient mice [56]. MyD88-deficient mice naturally display excess quantities of total IgE, because T cells from knockout (KO) mice release increased amounts of IL-13.

However, antigen-specific IgE responses were comparable between wild-type (WT) and KO mice that were immunized with alum plus OVA by footpad injection [56]. Furthermore, Gavin et al. also investigated alum adjuvanticity using MyD88 and Toll/IL-1 receptor domain-coding adaptor inducing IFN-γ (TRIF) double-KO mice, which completely lack TLR signaling. Similarly to MyD88 deficiency, the antibody responses were comparable between WT and double-KO mice immunized with trinitrophenol-hemocyanin plus alum by intraperitoneal injection [57]. However, Matsushita et al. demonstrated that B-cell-specific MyD88-deficient mice displayed reduced levels of serum antigen-specific IgE and IgG1 after the immunization with alum plus OVA through direct administration to the airway [58]. Thus, the requirement for MyD88 signaling might be dependent on the administration route and the specific cell type.

Several studies also demonstrated the requirement of MyD88 signaling in ambient air pollution particle-induced allergic responses. Becker et al. showed that microbial components on ambient particulate matter stimulate alveolar macrophage to produce inflammatory cytokines in a TLR4-dependent manner [59]. In addition, Ichinose et al. reported that microbial materials, in particular TLR2 ligands such as β-glucan and peptidoglycan, are involved in ASD-induced lung eosinophilia. ASD, to which LPS and β-glucan adhere, induced eosinophil infiltration in the lung; however this was reduced after heating of the ASD to exclude microbial components [60, 61]. In fact, TLR ligands are known to induce allergic lung inflammation [62], suggesting that ambient particulate adjuvant activates type-2 immune responses, in part, through TLR and MyD88 signaling promoted by microbial components adhered to the particulate.

Natural and synthetic hemozoin crystals that are not particulate adjuvants causing allergy also seem to activate MyD88 signaling which is required for adjuvant activity. The underlying mechanisms of the adjuvant activity of hemozoin remain to be investigated [49].

5.4.2 Inflammasome

The inflammasome is a type of intracellular PRR that is categorized into the NOD-like receptors. There are four classes of inflammasome, NLRP1, NLRP3, NLRC4 (IPAF), and AIM2, of which NLRP3 is the best characterized [24]. Upon activation, NLRP3 forms a multiprotein complex with apoptosis-associated speck-like protein containing a caspase recruitment domain (ASC) and caspase-1. This complex promotes the secretion of the pro-inflammatory cytokines IL-1β and IL-18 through the action of caspase-1 [24]. Initially, it was demonstrated that the NLRP3 inflammasome is activated by invasive infection and induces inflammatory responses [24]. Later in 2008, several reports demonstrated that particulates or crystals, such as silica, alum, and asbestos, stimulate macrophages and DCs to produce IL-1β and IL-18 through the activation of the NLRP3 inflammasome [63–65]. The NLRP3 inflammasome has been reported to be involved in type-2 immune responses, and in addition, alum-induced type-2 responses, especially IgG1 and IgE responses, are significantly reduced in NLRP3-, ASC-, and caspase-1-deficient mice. Interestingly, most particulate adjuvants activate the NLRP3 inflammasome in macrophages and DCs to produce mature IL-1β. For example, in addition to alum and silica, MSU acts as activator of the NLRP3 inflammasome [66]. Ambient particle pollutants, such as DEP, ASD, and PM2.5, are reported to stimulate innate cells to produce IL-1β and IL-18, implicating the importance of inflammasome activation [38, 67, 68]. In addition, PGLA and hydroxyapatite nanoparticles that do not induce allergic responses function as a vaccine adjuvant and induce IL-1β through the NLRP3 inflammasome [54, 55]. However, other reports have shown that the NLRP3 inflammasome is dispensable for adjuvant activity of particulates. In addition, it has been reported that the NLRP3 inflammasome is not required for antigen-specific antibody production induced by sensitization with alum plus antigens [69–71]. These contradictory reports on the role of the NLRP3 inflammasome indicate that further investigation is required to determine the importance of the inflammasome in particulate adjuvanticity. Inflammasome activation induced by particulates seems to be important for the induction of acute inflammation in the lung. Furthermore, several studies have shown that most inflammasome activators also induce IL-1α release from DCs, and particulate adjuvants such as alum, silica, MSU, and TiO$_2$ stimulate DCs to release IL-1α, a process that is partially dependent on the NLRP3 inflammasome [72, 73]. Another study also reported that IL-1α release was partially reduced in response to PGLA and polystyrene microparticles in DCs from NLRP3-deficient mice [54]. The detailed mechanism of inflammasome-dependent IL-1α release by particulate adjuvant is still unclear. Interestingly, a recent study demonstrated that IL-1α and IL-1β control inflammation at different stages, i.e., initiation and maintenance [74]. Thus, particulate adjuvants may regulate a many-sided immune response through NLRP3 inflammasome activation during inflammation. Recent reports have demonstrated a novel mechanism of inflammasome to perpetuate inflammatory responses [75, 76]. After the activation of inflammasome, ASC assembles into a large protein aggregate with NLRP3 and caspase-1. The inflammasome particles, or "specks," are released during pyroptotic cell death and taken up by surrounding phagocyte to lead to inflammation through the release of IL-1β. Thus, ASC speck acts as danger signals to spread inflammatory responses.

5.4.3 MSU Crystals

Uric acid is an intracellular purine catabolite that is released from dying or stressed cells. At saturated concentrations of uric acid, MSU crystals are formed. MSU crystals are considered as DAMPs that regulate immune responses at the site of inflammation, such as those that occur during gout. In 2003, Shi et al. demonstrated that uric acid and its crystals induce DC maturation and activation [77]. Interestingly, MSU crystals are reported to preferentially induce type-2 immune responses through their adjuvant activity. Kool et al. reported that levels of uric acid are increased in the peritoneal cavity after i.p. injection of alum. In addition, released uric acid seems to induce antigen-specific T-cell responses because administration of uricase significantly reduced the activation of T cells [12, 40]. Some particulates, such as alum and silica, are known to induce cell death. Furthermore, it is reported that ambient particle pollutants, PM2.5 and DEP, and metal-based nanoparticles also showed cytotoxic activity on macrophages and monocytes through the production of reactive oxygen species [78–80]. Given that particulates induce cell death, uric acid and MSU crystals released from dying cells by particulates might contribute to allergic inflammation. In fact, a recent study showed that allergic lung inflammation induced by the administration of airborne allergen to the airway is a uric acid- and IL-33-dependent mechanism and treatment with an inhibitor of uric acid synthesis attenuated the onset of asthma [43]. Kool et al. demonstrated that uric acid-primed inflammatory monocytes and DCs participate in T-cell activation through IL-1 and MyD88 signaling [40]. In addition, since uric acid (and its crystal form) is known to induce IL-1β through the activation of the NLRP3 inflammasome as described above, this adjuvant effect was considered to be dependent on IL-1β released by the activated inflammasome. However, it was reported that the NLRP3 inflammasome, IL-1, and MyD88 signaling are dispensable for the adjuvanticity of uric acid induced by alum [12, 14]. In addition, it was shown that spleen tyrosine kinase (Syk) and PI3-kinase δ in inflammatory monocytes and DCs participate in type-2 immune responses induced by uric acid [12]. So far, several papers have shown the importance of Syk in activation of macrophages and DCs. The underlying mechanisms of Syk activation by particulates and the role of Syk in type-2 immune responses are interesting issues that require further investigation [12, 14, 81]. Recent studies have reported the importance of Syk in immune responses induced by dead cells, demonstrating that Clec9a, one of the C-type lectin receptors (CLRs) in PRRs, senses necrotic cells and induces DC activation through the Syk-dependent signaling pathway [82, 83]. Several CLRs are coupled with Syk and transduce activating signals into cells [27]. Clec9a recognizes F-actin expressed on necrotic cells [82, 83]. Thus, Syk may play an important role in signal transduction for factors from dying cells.

The recognition mechanisms of MSU crystals have also been investigated. Ng et al. demonstrated that MSU crystals interact with the lipid raft on DCs in a receptor-independent manner. This interaction causes lipid sorting and transduces a signal into cells that then leads to recruitment and activation of Syk [81]. Flach et al. reported that alum also binds to the lipid raft on DCs and then activates Syk and PI3-kinase, similarly to MSU crystals. Then DCs activate T cells through the interaction with intracellular adhesion molecule (ICAM)-1 and leukocyte function-associated antigen (LFA)-1 [84].

5.4.4 Prostaglandin Production

Previously, we reported the unique function of particulates in eliciting type-2 immune responses. We focused on the particulates alum and silica and found that these particulates stimulated macrophages and DCs to produce the lipid mediator prostaglandin (PG), similar to the activation of the NLRP3 inflammasome [14].

PGE_2, a well-characterized pro-inflammatory lipid mediator, is an arachidonic acid metabolite that is mainly produced by myeloid-lineage cells such as DCs and macrophages [85]. PGE_2 performs various functions in the regulation of immune responses, one of which is the suppression of type-1 immune responses by inhibiting the production of type-1 cytokines such as IFN-γ and IL-12 [86–88].

Alum and silica stimulate LPS-primed macrophages and DCs to activate the NLRP3 inflammasome and release IL-1β and IL-18; in addition, we also observed PGE_2 release from particulate-activated macrophages and DCs. PGE_2 release was shown to be independent of the NLRP3 inflammasome and IL-1 signaling because inflammasome-deficient macrophages, such as NLRP3 KO, ASC KO, or caspase-1 KO macrophages, still produced normal levels of PGE_2 in response to alum and silica. Interestingly, PGE_2 production in response to alum and silica was mediated by the activation of Syk, which is an important molecule for the activation of DCs by MSU crystals. To clarify the role of PGE_2 in immune responses in vivo, we used PGE synthase (PTGES)-deficient mice [89]. Macrophages from PTGES-deficient mice did not produce PGE_2 in response to alum or silica. In addition, PTGES-deficient mice displayed reduced levels of antigen-specific IgE after immunization with alum + OVA or silica + OVA, indicating that particulate-induced PGE_2 regulates IgE production in vivo. Previous studies have shown that PGE_2 facilitates IgE production from B cells stimulated with IL-4, through the intracellular accumulation of cAMP [90, 91]. Furthermore, a recent study demonstrated that the elevated levels of PGE_2 in the gut are involved in allergic airway inflammation by the alteration of macrophage phenotypes toward type-2 macrophage (M2) [92].

We also found that many particulates such as MSU crystals, PGLA, nickel oxide, amorphous silica, and CNTs also stimulate macrophages to produce inflammasome-dependent IL-1β and inflammasome-independent PGE_2. In addition, increased amounts of PGE_2 release were observed in dying cells, indicating that, as with uric acid release, PGE_2 release is an indicator of cell death and might function as a DAMP (Kuroda et al. unpublished data). These results suggest that PGE_2 release in response to particulates is one of the markers of the adjuvanticity of particulates and may be a potent inducer of allergic inflammation.

5.4.5   Nucleic Acid

As described above, DAMP release in response to a particulate seems to be required for the induction of immune responses [28]. Recent studies have shown that a chemical agent that has cytotoxic activity acts as an adjuvant to induce IgE production, suggesting that particulate-induced DAMPs may participate in allergic inflammation [93, 94]. DNA released from host cells appears to be a DAMP. Marichal et al. demonstrated that DNA from damaged host cells is involved in the adjuvanticity of alum [16]. This study showed that host DNA is released from damaged phagocytes such as macrophage and neutrophils at the site of alum injection. The released DNA functions as an adjuvant and induces antigen-specific IgG and IgE responses. Interestingly, treatment with DNase I at the injection site of alum + OVA significantly reduced OVA-specific antibody responses. In addition, purified genomic DNA mixed with antigen mimicked the adjuvant activity of alum and induced antigen-specific antibody responses. This finding indicates that DNA released from host cells is a critical factor for the activation of innate and adaptive immune responses. TANK-binding kinase 1(TBK-1) and interferon regulatory factor 3 (IRF-3) are reported to be important signaling molecules downstream of specific receptors for DNA recognition in innate cells [95]. This study demonstrated the attenuated adjuvant activities of alum or host DNA in TBK1- or IRF3-deficient mice, with IgE responses being markedly reduced. In addition, IRF3 participates in the recruitment of inflammatory monocytes and DCs, cells responsible for the induction of type-2 immune responses, suggesting that IRF3 regulates the type-2 adjuvant activity of alum through the signaling pathway for host DNA recognition during an innate immune response. The IRF3-mediated activation of inflammatory DCs was controlled by IL-12p80 release, a p40 homodimer. Furthermore, treatment of IL-12p80 neutralizing antibody partially reduced IgE responses in mice immunized with alum + OVA. Given that many particulates with adjuvant activity are known to induce cell death, the adjuvant activity of particulates is considered to be closely linked to cell death and consequently host DNA release. CpG oligodeoxynucleotide is a well-known DNA-based adjuvant that is recognized by TLR9, but it is reported to be a strong inducer of type-1 immunity unlike the DNA released from dying cells [96, 97], suggesting that different types of DNA induce type-2 immune responses through signal transduction pathways other than TLR9 signaling.

A recent study demonstrated that DNA released from damaged cells directly stimulates naive CD4+ T cells to induce Th2 differentiation through an unknown DNA sensor and might be involved in allergic inflammation [98]. The underlying mechanisms for Th2 differentiation were mediated by the downregulation of T-bet and the upregulation of GATA-3 expression. Furthermore, a recently identified DNA sensor, cyclic GMP-AMP synthase (cGAS), might be important for type-2 immunity [99]. Activated cGAS induces generation of cyclic AMP-GMP (cGAMP), and this cyclic nucleotide functions as the ligand for the ER-resident adaptor molecules, stimulator of interferon genes (STING). Activated STING is known to regulate the TBK1-IRF3 signaling pathway to induce type-1 IFN production [100, 101]. Our previous studies demonstrated that cGAMP and synthetic STING ligand function as type-2 adjuvants and induce antigen-specific Th2 responses [102, 103]. Interestingly, STING ligand-induced type-2 responses were IRF3 and type-1 IFN dependent and were completely abolished in IRF3- and type-1 IFN receptor-deficient mice [102, 103]. Given that IRF3 and TBK1 are involved in host DNA-dependent adjuvant activity by alum, these signaling molecules may be potent therapeutic targets of particulate-induced allergic inflammation. Thus, host DNA and DNA-sensing molecule and its signal transducers appear to augment allergic inflammation through both known and unknown mechanisms.

It is not only DNA that is released from damaged cells; uric acid and its crystals are also released. We also found that higher levels of PGE_2 were released during cell death (unpublished data). Taken together, it is evident that many different types of DAMPs released from dying cells induced by particulates promote immune responses and exacerbate allergic inflammation.

5.5   Th2 Cytokine-Producing Cells

Particulate adjuvants including particle pollutants promote antigen (allergen)-specific IgE, and in general Th2 cytokines IL-4 or IL-13 and signal transducer and activator of transcription 6 (STAT6) are required for class switching to IgE in B cells. In fact, Brewer et al. demonstrated that serum IgE production was abolished in IL-4 receptor- and STAT6-deficient mice immunized with antigen + alum [104, 105]. However, the question of how alum induces IL-4-producing cells has remained poorly studied. Several reports observed IL-4-producing cells after the administration of alum. Jordan et al. showed that Gr-1+ IL-4-producing cells were recruited to the injection site of alum, and Wang et al. confirmed that the alum-elicited IL-4-producing cells were eosinophils and basophils [106, 107]. Furthermore, chitin particles, which are potent allergic inflammation inducers, also promote the recruitment of IL-4-producing cells that are identified as eosinophils and basophils [17]. However, it has been reported that IgE responses are normal in both eosinophil-deficient and basophil-deficient mice that are immunized with OVA + alum [69, 108]. A recent study has demonstrated that type-2, but not type-1, natural killer T (NKT) cells appear to be required for alum-induced antibody responses by the regulation of IL-4-producing T cells [109].

Recently, unique cells have been reported to play a role in the regulation of IgE production and Th2 differentiation, namely, group 2 innate lymphoid cells (ILC2) [110, 111]. ILC2 cells were identified by three different research groups as "natural helper cells," "nuocytes," or "innate helper 2 cells" [112–114]. ILC2 cells produce higher amounts of IL-5 and IL-13 in response to IL-25 and IL-33 and play an important role in protective immunity against helminth infection. In addition, recent studies have demonstrated that ILC2 cells also regulate Th2 differentiation using a protein allergen-induced lung inflammation model [115, 116]. So far, there is no clear evidence whether or not particulate adjuvants stimulate ILC2 cells, but this question may be solved in the near future. Another unique cell type is follicular helper T (Tfh) cells [117]. Tfh cells were identified as a subset of germinal center (GC) CD4+ T cells that differ from conventional Th2 cells [118–121]. Tfh cells are reported to produce IL-4 in GC and are considered a critical source of IL-4 for IgE production [122]. In fact, recent studies have shown that mice that are specifically deficient in IL-4 production by Tfh cells, but not Th2 cells, displayed a significant reduction in IgG1 and IgE after the immunization with antigen + alum; however differentiation into Th2 cells and IL-4 production was normal in these deficient mice [123, 124]. These results might imply that particulate adjuvants preferentially activate Tfh cells to produce IL-4, in a cell death-dependent manner.

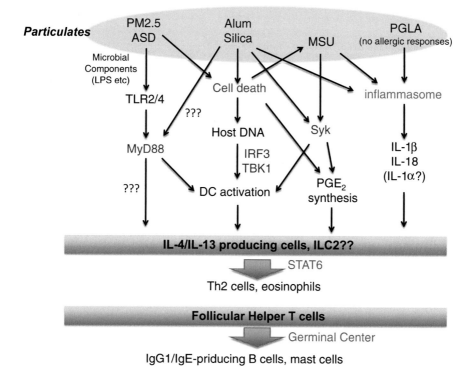

Fig. 5.2 Summary of proposed models of the mechanism of action of particulate adjuvant. Particulate adjuvants induce immune responses through TLR signaling, inflammasome activation, or DAMP release from damaged cells

5.6 Conclusion

We summarized the mechanism of action of particulate causing allergy in the immune system in Fig. 5.2. In this review, we focused on the effect of particulate adjuvants on allergic inflammation. To date, many studies have demonstrated that some kind of particulates induce and exacerbate allergic inflammation as characterized by the activation of eosinophils and the induction of serum IgE. However, the mechanistic details remain to be determined, as does the mode of action of alum despite the fact that alum has been extensively employed as a human vaccine adjuvant. Advances in particulate adjuvant research could open new possibilities for the treatment of particulate-induced allergic disorders.

Declaration of Interest EK received a Grant-in-Aid for Scientific Research from the Ministry of Education, Culture, Sports, Science and Technology (MEXT) of Japan (grant number 24591145 and 15K15390) and Takeda Science Foundation and the Mochida Memorial Foundation for Medical and Pharmaceutical Research. KJI and CC were supported by a Health and Labor Science Research Grant "Adjuvant Database Project" from the Japan Agency for Medical Research and Development (AMED).

References

1. Bartra J, Mullol J, del Cuvillo A, Davila I, Ferrer M, Jauregui I, et al. Air pollution and allergens. J Investig Allergol Clin Immunol. 2007;17 Suppl 2:3–8.
2. Granum B, Gaarder PI, Groeng E, Leikvold R, Namork E, Lovik M. Fine particles of widely different composition have an adjuvant effect on the production of allergen-specific antibodies. Toxicol Lett. 2001;118(3):171–81.
3. Hiyoshi K, Ichinose T, Sadakane K, Takano H, Nishikawa M, Mori I, et al. Asian sand dust enhances ovalbumin-induced eosinophil recruitment in the alveoli and airway of mice. Environ Res. 2005;99(3):361–8. doi:10.1016/j.envres.2005.03.008.
4. Honda A, Matsuda Y, Murayama R, Tsuji K, Nishikawa M, Koike E, et al. Effects of Asian sand dust particles on the respiratory and immune system. JAT. 2014;34(3):250–7. doi:10.1002/jat.2871.
5. Ichinose T, Takano H, Miyabara Y, Yanagisawa R, Sagai M. Murine strain differences in allergic airway inflammation and immunoglobulin production by a combination of antigen and diesel exhaust particles. Toxicology. 1997;122(3):183–92.
6. Inoue K, Koike E, Yanagisawa R, Hirano S, Nishikawa M, Takano H. Effects of multi-walled carbon nanotubes on a murine allergic airway inflammation model. Toxicol Appl Pharmacol. 2009;237(3):306–16. doi:10.1016/j.taap.2009.04.003.
7. Lovik M, Hogseth AK, Gaarder PI, Hagemann R, Eide I. Diesel exhaust particles and carbon black have adjuvant activity on the local lymph node response and systemic IgE production to ovalbumin. Toxicology. 1997;121(2):165–78.
8. Nygaard UC, Hansen JS, Samuelsen M, Alberg T, Marioara CD, Lovik M. Single-walled and multi-walled carbon nanotubes promote allergic immune responses in mice. Toxicol Sci. 2009;109(1):113–23. doi:10.1093/toxsci/kfp057.
9. Ueda K, Nitta H, Odajima H. The effects of weather, air pollutants, and Asian dust on hospitalization for asthma in Fukuoka. Environ Health Prev Med. 2010;15(6):350–7. doi:10.1007/s12199-010-0150-5.
10. Schwartz J, Slater D, Larson TV, Pierson WE, Koenig JQ. Particulate air pollution and hospital emergency room visits for asthma in Seattle. Am Rev Respir Dis. 1993;147(4):826–31. doi:10.1164/ajrccm/147.4.826.
11. Pulendran B, Artis D. New paradigms in type 2 immunity. Science. 2012;337(6093):431–5. doi:10.1126/science.1221064.
12. Kool M, Willart MA, van Nimwegen M, Bergen I, Pouliot P, Virchow JC, et al. An unexpected role for uric acid as an inducer of T helper 2 cell immunity to inhaled antigens and inflammatory mediator of allergic asthma. Immunity. 2011;34(4):527–40. doi:10.1016/j.immuni.2011.03.015.
13. Kuroda E, Coban C, Ishii KJ. Particulate adjuvant and innate immunity: past achievements, present findings, and future prospects. Int Rev Immunol. 2013;32(2):209–20. doi:10.3109/08830185.2013.773326.
14. Kuroda E, Ishii KJ, Uematsu S, Ohata K, Coban C, Akira S, et al. Silica crystals and aluminum salts regulate the production of prostaglandin in macrophages via NALP3 inflammasome-independent mechanisms. Immunity. 2011;34(4):514–26. doi:10.1016/j.immuni.2011.03.019.
15. Mancino D, Buono G, Cusano M, Minucci M. Adjuvant effects of a crystalline silica on IgE and IgG1 antibody production in mice and their prevention by the macrophage stabilizer poly-2-vinylpyridine N-oxide. Int Arch Allergy Appl Immunol. 1983;71(3):279–81.
16. Marichal T, Ohata K, Bedoret D, Mesnil C, Sabatel C, Kobiyama K, et al. DNA released from dying host cells mediates aluminum adjuvant activity. Nat Med. 2011;17(8):996–1002. doi:10.1038/nm.2403.
17. Reese TA, Liang HE, Tager AM, Luster AD, Van Rooijen N, Voehringer D, et al. Chitin induces accumulation in tissue of innate immune cells associated with allergy. Nature. 2007;447(7140):92–6. doi:10.1038/nature05746.

18. Gupta RK. Aluminum compounds as vaccine adjuvants. Adv Drug Deliv Rev. 1998;32:155–72. doi:S0169-409X(98)00008-8 [pii].

19. Aimanianda V, Haensler J, Lacroix-Desmazes S, Kaveri SV, Bayry J. Novel cellular and molecular mechanisms of induction of immune responses by aluminum adjuvants. Trends Pharmacol Sci. 2009;30:287–95. doi:10.1016/j.tips.2009.03.005. doi:S0165-6147(09)00067-4 [pii].

20. Marrack P, McKee AS, Munks MW. Towards an understanding of the adjuvant action of aluminium. Nat Rev Immunol. 2009;9:287–93. doi:10.1038/nri2510. doi:nri2510 [pii].

21. Akira S. Innate immunity and adjuvants. Philos Trans R Soc B. 2011;366:2748–55. doi:10.1098/rstb.2011.0106.

22. Iwasaki A, Medzhitov R. Regulation of adaptive immunity by the innate immune system. Science. 2010;327:291–5. doi:10.1126/science.1183021. 327/5963/291 [pii].

23. Coquerelle C, Moser M. DC subsets in positive and negative regulation of immunity. Immunol Rev. 2010;234:317–34. doi:10.1111/j.0105-2896.2009.00887.x. IMR887 [pii].

24. Elinav E, Strowig T, Henao-Mejia J, Flavell RA. Regulation of the antimicrobial response by NLR proteins. Immunity. 2011;34:665–79. doi:10.1016/j.immuni.2011.05.007.

25. Kawai T, Akira S. Toll-like receptors and their crosstalk with other innate receptors in infection and immunity. Immunity. 2011;34:637–50. doi:10.1016/j.immuni.2011.05.006.

26. Loo Y-M, Gale M. Immune signaling by RIG-I-like receptors. Immunity. 2011;34:680–92. doi:10.1016/j.immuni.2011.05.003.

27. Osorio F, Reis e Sousa C. Myeloid C-type lectin receptors in pathogen recognition and host defense. Immunity. 2011;34:651–64. doi:10.1016/j.immuni.2011.05.001.

28. Desmet CJ, Ishii KJ. Nucleic acid sensing at the interface between innate and adaptive immunity in vaccination. Nat Rev Immunol. 2012;12:479–91. doi:10.1038/nri3247. nri3247 [pii].

29. Ghaemi-Oskouie F, Shi Y. The role of uric acid as an endogenous danger signal in immunity and inflammation. Curr Rheumatol Rep. 2011;13(2):160–6. doi:10.1007/s11926-011-0162-1.

30. Jounai N, Kobiyama K, Takeshita F, Ishii KJ. Recognition of damage-associated molecular patterns related to nucleic acids during inflammation and vaccination. Front Cell Infect Microbiol. 2012;2:168. doi:10.3389/fcimb.2012.00168.

31. Kono H, Chen CJ, Ontiveros F, Rock KL. Uric acid promotes an acute inflammatory response to sterile cell death in mice. J Clin Invest. 2010;120(6):1939–49. doi:10.1172/JCI40124.

32. Said-Sadier N, Ojcius DM. Alarmins, inflammasomes and immunity. Biomed J. 2012;35(6):437–49. doi:10.4103/2319-4170.104408.

33. Shen H, Kreisel D, Goldstein DR. Processes of sterile inflammation. J Immunol. 2013;191(6):2857–63. doi:10.4049/jimmunol.1301539.

34. Willart MA, Lambrecht BN. The danger within: endogenous danger signals, atopy and asthma. Clin Exp Allergy. 2009;39(1):12–9. doi:10.1111/j.1365-2222.2008.03118.x.

35. Rock KL, Lai JJ, Kono H. Innate and adaptive immune responses to cell death. Immunol Rev. 2011;243(1):191–205. doi:10.1111/j.1600-065X.2011.01040.x.

36. Bianchi ME. DAMPs, PAMPs and alarmins: all we need to know about danger. J Leukoc Biol. 2007;81(1):1–5. doi:10.1189/jlb.0306164.

37. Zhang X, Zhong W, Meng Q, Lin Q, Fang C, Huang X, et al. Ambient PM2.5 exposure exacerbates severity of allergic asthma in previously sensitized mice. J Asthma. 2015;52(8):785–94. doi:10.3109/02770903.2015.1036437.

38. Ogino K, Zhang R, Takahashi H, Takemoto K, Kubo M, Murakami I, et al. Allergic airway inflammation by nasal inoculation of particulate matter (PM2.5) in NC/Nga mice. PLoS One. 2014;9(3):e92710. doi:10.1371/journal.pone.0092710.

39. Williams GR, Fierens K, Preston SG, Lunn D, Rysnik O, De Prijck S, et al. Immunity induced by a broad class of inorganic crystalline materials is directly controlled by their chemistry. J Exp Med. 2014;211(6):1019–25. doi:10.1084/jem.20131768.

40. Kool M, Soullie T, van Nimwegen M, Willart MAM, Muskens F, Jung S, et al. Alum adjuvant boosts adaptive immunity by inducing uric acid and activating inflammatory dendritic cells. J Exp Med. 2008;205:869–82. doi:10.1084/jem.20071087.
41. Behrens MD, Wagner WM, Krco CJ, Erskine CL, Kalli KR, Krempski J, et al. The endogenous danger signal, crystalline uric acid, signals for enhanced antibody immunity. Blood. 2008;111:1472–9. doi:10.1182/blood-2007-10-117184. doi:blood-2007-10-117184 [pii].
42. Kool M, Hammad H, Lambrecht B. Cellular networks controlling Th2 polarization in allergy and immunity. F1000. Biol Rep. 2012;4:6. doi:10.3410/b4-6.
43. Hara K, Iijima K, Elias MK, Seno S, Tojima I, Kobayashi T, et al. Airway uric acid is a sensor of inhaled protease allergens and initiates type 2 immune responses in respiratory mucosa. J Immunol. 2014;192(9):4032–42. doi:10.4049/jimmunol.1400110.
44. Muller J, Huaux F, Moreau N, Misson P, Heilier JF, Delos M, et al. Respiratory toxicity of multi-wall carbon nanotubes. Toxicol Appl Pharmacol. 2005;207(3):221–31. doi:10.1016/j. taap.2005.01.008.
45. Shvedova AA, Kisin ER, Mercer R, Murray AR, Johnson VJ, Potapovich AI, et al. Unusual inflammatory and fibrogenic pulmonary responses to single-walled carbon nanotubes in mice. Am J Physiol Lung Cell Mol Physiol. 2005;289(5):L698–708. doi:10.1152/ ajplung.00084.2005.
46. Nilsen A, Hagemann R, Eide I. The adjuvant activity of diesel exhaust particles and carbon black on systemic IgE production to ovalbumin in mice after intranasal instillation. Toxicology. 1997;124(3):225–32.
47. de Haar C, Hassing I, Bol M, Bleumink R, Pieters R. Ultrafine carbon black particles cause early airway inflammation and have adjuvant activity in a mouse allergic airway disease model. Toxicol Sci. 2005;87(2):409–18. doi:10.1093/toxsci/kfi255.
48. Inoue K, Takano H, Yanagisawa R, Sakurai M, Ichinose T, Sadakane K, et al. Effects of nano particles on antigen-related airway inflammation in mice. Respir Res. 2005;6:106. doi:10.1186/1465-9921-6-106.
49. Coban C, Igari Y, Yagi M, Reimer T, Koyama S, Aoshi T, et al. Immunogenicity of whole-parasite vaccines against plasmodium falciparum involves malarial hemozoin and host TLR9. Cell Host Microbe. 2010;7:50–61. doi:10.1016/j.chom.2009.12.003.
50. Coban C, Yagi M, Ohata K, Igari Y, Tsukui T, Horii T, et al. The malarial metabolite hemozoin and its potential use as a vaccine adjuvant. Allergol Int. 2010;59:115–24. doi:10.2332/ allergolint.10-RAI-0194. 059020115 [pii].
51. Onishi M, Kitano M, Taniguchi K, Homma T, Kobayashi M, Sato A, et al. Hemozoin is a potent adjuvant for hemagglutinin split vaccine without pyrogenicity in ferrets. Vaccine. 2014;32(25):3004–9. doi:10.1016/j.vaccine.2014.03.072.
52. Uraki R, Das SC, Hatta M, Kiso M, Iwatsuki-Horimoto K, Ozawa M, et al. Hemozoin as a novel adjuvant for inactivated whole virion influenza vaccine. Vaccine. 2014;32(41):5295– 300. doi:10.1016/j.vaccine.2014.07.079.
53. Akagi T, Baba M, Akashi M. Biodegradable nanoparticles as vaccine adjuvants and delivery systems: regulation of immune responses by nanoparticle-based vaccine. Adv Polym Sci. 2011;247:31–64. doi:10.1007/12_2011_150.
54. Sharp FA, Ruane D, Claass B, Creagh E, Harris J, Malyala P, et al. Uptake of particulate vaccine adjuvants by dendritic cells activates the NALP3 inflammasome. Proc Natl Acad Sci U S A. 2009;106(3):870–5. doi:10.1073/pnas.0804897106.
55. Hayashi M, Aoshi T, Kogai Y, Nomi D, Haseda Y, Kuroda E, et al. Optimization of physiological properties of hydroxyapatite as a vaccine adjuvant. Vaccine. 2016;34(3):306–12. doi:10.1016/j.vaccine.2015.11.059.
56. Schnare M, Barton GM, Holt AC, Takeda K, Akira S, Medzhitov R. Toll-like receptors control activation of adaptive immune responses. Nat Immunol. 2001;2:947–50. doi:10.1038/ ni712. ni712 [pii].
57. Gavin AL, Hoebe K, Duong B, Ota T, Martin C, Beutler B, et al. Adjuvant-enhanced antibody responses in the absence of toll-like receptor signaling. Science. 2006;314:1936–8. doi:10.1126/science.1135299.

58. Matsushita K, Yoshimoto T. B cell-intrinsic MyD88 signaling is essential for IgE responses in lungs exposed to pollen allergens. J Immunol. 2014;193(12):5791–800. doi:10.4049/jimmunol.1401768.

59. Becker S, Fenton MJ, Soukup JM. Involvement of microbial components and toll-like receptors 2 and 4 in cytokine responses to air pollution particles. Am J Respir Cell Mol Biol. 2002;27(5):611–8. doi:10.1165/rcmb.4868.

60. Ichinose T, Yoshida S, Hiyoshi K, Sadakane K, Takano H, Nishikawa M, et al. The effects of microbial materials adhered to Asian sand dust on allergic lung inflammation. Arch Environ Contam Toxicol. 2008;55(3):348–57. doi:10.1007/s00244-007-9128-8.

61. Ren Y, Ichinose T, He M, Song Y, Yoshida Y, Yoshida S, et al. Enhancement of OVA-induced murine lung eosinophilia by co-exposure to contamination levels of LPS in Asian sand dust and heated dust. Allergy Asthma Clin Immunol. 2014;10(1):30. doi:10.1186/1710-1492-10-30.

62. Reuter S, Dehzad N, Martin H, Bohm L, Becker M, Buhl R, et al. TLR3 but not TLR7/8 ligand induces allergic sensitization to inhaled allergen. J Immunol. 2012;188(10):5123–31. doi:10.4049/jimmunol.1101618.

63. Eisenbarth SC, Colegio OR, O'Connor W, Sutterwala FS, Flavell RA. Crucial role for the Nalp3 inflammasome in the immunostimulatory properties of aluminium adjuvants. Nature. 2008;453:1122–6. doi:10.1038/nature06939.

64. Hornung V, Bauernfeind F, Halle A, Samstad EO, Kono H, Rock KL, et al. Silica crystals and aluminum salts activate the NALP3 inflammasome through phagosomal destabilization. Nat Immunol. 2008;9:847–56. doi:10.1038/ni.1631. doi:ni.1631 [pii].

65. Dostert C, Petrilli V, Van Bruggen R, Steele C, Mossman BT, Tschopp J. Innate immune activation through Nalp3 inflammasome sensing of asbestos and silica. Science. 2008;320:674–7. doi:10.1126/science.1156995.

66. Martinon F, Petrilli V, Mayor A, Tardivel A, Tschopp J. Gout-associated uric acid crystals activate the NALP3 inflammasome. Nature. 2006;440:237–41. doi:10.1038/nature04516. doi:nature04516 [pii].

67. He M, Ichinose T, Yoshida S, Yamamoto S, Inoue K, Takano H, et al. Asian sand dust enhances murine lung inflammation caused by Klebsiella pneumoniae. Toxicol Appl Pharmacol. 2012;258(2):237–47. doi:10.1016/j.taap.2011.11.003.

68. Ather JL, Martin RA, Ckless K, Poynter ME. Inflammasome activity in non-microbial lung inflammation. J Environ Immunol Toxicol. 2014;1(3):108–17.

69. McKee AS, Munks MW, MacLeod MKL, Fleenor CJ, Van Rooijen N, Kappler JW, et al. Alum induces innate immune responses through macrophage and mast cell sensors, but these sensors are not required for alum to act as an adjuvant for specific immunity. J Immunol. 2009;183:4403–14. doi:10.4049/jimmunol.0900164.

70. Kool M, Petrilli V, De Smedt T, Rolaz A, Hammad H, van Nimwegen M, et al. Cutting edge: alum adjuvant stimulates inflammatory dendritic cells through activation of the NALP3 inflammasome. J Immunol. 2008;181:3755–9. doi:181/6/3755 [pii].

71. Franchi L, Núñez G. The Nlrp3 inflammasome is critical for aluminium hydroxide-mediated IL-1β secretion but dispensable for adjuvant activity. Eur J Immunol. 2008;38:2085–9. doi:10.1002/eji.200838549.

72. Yazdi AS, Guarda G, Riteau N, Drexler SK, Tardivel A, Couillin I, et al. Nanoparticles activate the NLR pyrin domain containing 3 (Nlrp3) inflammasome and cause pulmonary inflammation through release of IL-1alpha and IL-1beta. Proc Natl Acad Sci U S A. 2010;107(45):19449–54. doi:10.1073/pnas.1008155107.

73. Gross O, Yazdi AS, Thomas CJ, Masin M, Heinz LX, Guarda G, et al. Inflammasome activators induce interleukin-1alpha secretion via distinct pathways with differential requirement for the protease function of caspase-1. Immunity. 2012;36(3):388–400. doi:10.1016/j.immuni.2012.01.018.

74. Rider P, Carmi Y, Guttman O, Braiman A, Cohen I, Voronov E, et al. IL-1alpha and IL-1beta recruit different myeloid cells and promote different stages of sterile inflammation. J Immunol. 2011;187(9):4835–43. doi:10.4049/jimmunol.1102048.

75. Franklin BS, Bossaller L, De Nardo D, Ratter JM, Stutz A, Engels G, et al. The adaptor ASC has extracellular and 'prionoid' activities that propagate inflammation. Nat Immunol. 2014;15(8):727–37. doi:10.1038/ni.2913.

76. Baroja-Mazo A, Martin-Sanchez F, Gomez AI, Martinez CM, Amores-Iniesta J, Compan V, et al. The NLRP3 inflammasome is released as a particulate danger signal that amplifies the inflammatory response. Nat Immunol. 2014;15(8):738–48. doi:10.1038/ni.2919.

77. Shi Y, Evans JE, Rock KL. Molecular identification of a danger signal that alerts the immune system to dying cells. Nature. 2003;425:516–21. doi:10.1038/nature01991. nature01991 [pii].

78. Yan B, Li J, Guo J, Ma P, Wu Z, Ling Z, et al. The toxic effects of indoor atmospheric fine particulate matter collected from allergic and non-allergic families in Wuhan on mouse peritoneal macrophages. JAT. 2015. doi:10.1002/jat.3217.

79. Hiura TS, Kaszubowski MP, Li N, Nel AE. Chemicals in diesel exhaust particles generate reactive oxygen radicals and induce apoptosis in macrophages. J Immunol. 1999;163(10):5582–91.

80. Petrarca C, Clemente E, Amato V, Pedata P, Sabbioni E, Bernardini G, et al. Engineered metal based nanoparticles and innate immunity. Clin Mol Allergy. 2015;13(1):13. doi:10.1186/s12948-015-0020-1.

81. Ng G, Sharma K, Ward SM, Desrosiers MD, Stephens LA, Schoel WM, et al. Receptor-independent, direct membrane binding leads to cell-surface lipid sorting and Syk kinase activation in dendritic cells. Immunity. 2008;29:807–18. doi:10.1016/j.immuni.2008.09.013. doi:S1074-7613(08)00463-9 [pii].

82. Ahrens S, Zelenay S, Sancho D, Hanc P, Kjaer S, Feest C, et al. F-actin is an evolutionarily conserved damage-associated molecular pattern recognized by DNGR-1, a receptor for dead cells. Immunity. 2012;36(4):635–45. doi:10.1016/j.immuni.2012.03.008.

83. Zhang JG, Czabotar PE, Policheni AN, Caminschi I, Wan SS, Kitsoulis S, et al. The dendritic cell receptor Clec9A binds damaged cells via exposed actin filaments. Immunity. 2012;36(4):646–57. doi:10.1016/j.immuni.2012.03.009.

84. Flach TL, Ng G, Hari A, Desrosiers MD, Zhang P, Ward SM, et al. Alum interaction with dendritic cell membrane lipids is essential for its adjuvanticity. Nat Med. 2011;17:479–87. doi:10.1038/nm.2306.

85. Narumiya S. Prostanoids and inflammation: a new concept arising from receptor knockout mice. J Mol Med (Berl). 2009;87:1015–22. doi:10.1007/s00109-009-0500-1.

86. Fabricius D, Neubauer M, Mandel B, Schutz C, Viardot A, Vollmer A, et al. Prostaglandin E2 inhibits IFN-alpha secretion and Th1 costimulation by human plasmacytoid dendritic cells via E-prostanoid 2 and E-prostanoid 4 receptor engagement. J Immunol. 2010;184:677–84. doi:10.4049/jimmunol.0902028. doi:jimmunol.0902028 [pii].

87. Kuroda E, Yamashita U. Mechanisms of enhanced macrophage-mediated prostaglandin E2 production and its suppressive role in Th1 activation in Th2-dominant BALB/c mice. J Immunol. 2003;170:757–64.

88. Koga K, Takaesu G, Yoshida R, Nakaya M, Kobayashi T, Kinjyo I, et al. Cyclic adenosine monophosphate suppresses the transcription of proinflammatory cytokines via the phosphorylated c-Fos protein. Immunity. 2009;30:372–83. doi:10.1016/j.immuni.2008.12.021. doi:S1074-7613(09)00103-4 [pii].

89. Uematsu S, Matsumoto M, Takeda K, Akira S. Lipopolysaccharide-dependent prostaglandin E(2) production is regulated by the glutathione-dependent prostaglandin E(2) synthase gene induced by the toll-like receptor 4/MyD88/NF-IL6 pathway. J Immunol. 2002;168:5811–6.

90. Fedyk ER, Phipps RP. Prostaglandin E2 receptors of the EP2 and EP4 subtypes regulate activation and differentiation of mouse B lymphocytes to IgE-secreting cells. Proc Natl Acad Sci U S A. 1996;93:10978–83.

91. Roper RL, Brown DM, Phipps RP. Prostaglandin E2 promotes B lymphocyte Ig isotype switching to IgE. J Immunol. 1995;154:162–70.

92. Kim YG, Udayanga KG, Totsuka N, Weinberg JB, Nunez G, Shibuya A. Gut dysbiosis promotes M2 macrophage polarization and allergic airway inflammation via fungi-induced PGE(2). Cell Host Microbe. 2014;15(1):95–102. doi:10.1016/j.chom.2013.12.010.

93. Jacobson LS, Lima Jr H, Goldberg MF, Gocheva V, Tsiperson V, Sutterwala FS, et al. Cathepsin-mediated necrosis controls the adaptive immune response by Th2 (T helper type 2)-associated adjuvants. J Biol Chem. 2013;288(11):7481–91. doi:10.1074/jbc.M112.400655.

94. Tonti E, Oya N, Galliverti G, Moseman EA, Di Lucia P, Amabile A, et al. Bisphosphonates target B cells to enhance humoral immune responses. Cell Rep. 2013;5(2):323–30. 1016/j. celrep.2013.09.004.

95. Ishii KJ, Kawagoe T, Koyama S, Matsui K, Kumar H, Kawai T, et al. TANK-binding kinase-1 delineates innate and adaptive immune responses to DNA vaccines. Nature. 2008;451(7179):725–9. doi:10.1038/nature06537.

96. Kawai T, Akira S. The role of pattern-recognition receptors in innate immunity: update on Toll-like receptors. Nat Immunol. 2010;11(5):373–84. doi:10.1038/ni.1863.

97. Krieg AM. Therapeutic potential of toll-like receptor 9 activation. Nat Rev Drug Discov. 2006;5(6):471–84. doi:10.1038/nrd2059.

98. Imanishi T, Ishihara C, Badr Mel S, Hashimoto-Tane A, Kimura Y, Kawai T, et al. Nucleic acid sensing by T cells initiates Th2 cell differentiation. Nat Commun. 2014;5:3566. doi:10.1038/ncomms4566.

99. Li XD, Wu J, Gao D, Wang H, Sun L, Chen ZJ. Pivotal roles of cGAS-cGAMP signaling in antiviral defense and immune adjuvant effects. Science. 2013;341(6152):1390–4. doi:10.1126/science.1244040.

100. Burdette DL, Monroe KM, Sotelo-Troha K, Iwig JS, Eckert B, Hyodo M, et al. STING is a direct innate immune sensor of cyclic di-GMP. Nature. 2011;478(7370):515–8. doi:10.1038/nature10429.

101. McWhirter SM, Barbalat R, Monroe KM, Fontana MF, Hyodo M, Joncker NT, et al. A host type I interferon response is induced by cytosolic sensing of the bacterial second messenger cyclic-di-GMP. J Exp Med. 2009;206(9):1899–911. doi:10.1084/jem.20082874.

102. Tang CK, Aoshi T, Jounai N, Ito J, Ohata K, Kobiyama K, et al. The chemotherapeutic agent DMXAA as a unique IRF3-dependent type-2 vaccine adjuvant. PLoS One. 2013;8(3):e60038. doi:10.1371/journal.pone.0060038.

103. Temizoz B, Kuroda E, Ohata K, Jounai N, Ozasa K, Kobiyama K, et al. TLR9 and STING agonists synergistically induce innate and adaptive type-II IFN. Eur J Immunol. 2015;45(4):1159–69. doi:10.1002/eji.201445132.

104. Brewer JM, Conacher M, Hunter CA, Mohrs M, Brombacher F, Alexander J. Aluminium hydroxide adjuvant initiates strong antigen-specific Th2 responses in the absence of IL-4- or IL-13-mediated signaling. J Immunol. 1999;163:6448–54. doi:ji_v163n12p6448 [pii].

105. Brewer JM, Conacher M, Satoskar A, Bluethmann H, Alexander J. In interleukin-4-deficient mice, alum not only generates T helper 1 responses equivalent to freund's complete adjuvant, but continues to induce T helper 2 cytokine production. Eur J Immunol. 1996;26:2062–6. doi:10.1002/eji.1830260915.

106. Jordan MB. Promotion of B cell immune responses via an alum-induced myeloid cell population. Science. 2004;304(5678):1808–10. doi:10.1126/science.1089926.

107. Wang HB, Weller PF. Pivotal advance: eosinophils mediate early alum adjuvant-elicited B cell priming and IgM production. J Leukoc Biol. 2008;83:817–21. doi:10.1189/jlb.0607392.

108. Ohnmacht C, Schwartz C, Panzer M, Schiedewitz I, Naumann R, Voehringer D. Basophils orchestrate chronic allergic dermatitis and protective immunity against helminths. Immunity. 2010;33:364–74. doi:10.1016/j.immuni.2010.08.011. doi:S1074-7613(10)00316-X [pii].

109. Shah HB, Devera TS, Rampuria P, Lang GA, Lang ML. Type II NKT cells facilitate alum-sensing and humoral immunity. J Leukoc Biol. 2012;92:883–93. doi:10.1189/jlb.0412177.

110. Licona-Limon P, Kim LK, Palm NW, Flavell RA. Th2, allergy and group 2 innate lymphoid cells. Nat Immunol. 2013;14(6):536–42. doi:10.1038/ni.2617.

111. Artis D, Spits H. The biology of innate lymphoid cells. Nature. 2015;517(7534):293–301. doi:10.1038/nature14189.

112. Moro K, Yamada T, Tanabe M, Takeuchi T, Ikawa T, Kawamoto H, et al. Innate production of T(H)2 cytokines by adipose tissue-associated c-Kit(+)Sca-1(+) lymphoid cells. Nature. 2010;463(7280):540–4. doi:10.1038/nature08636.

113. Neill DR, Wong SH, Bellosi A, Flynn RJ, Daly M, Langford TK, et al. Nuocytes represent a new innate effector leukocyte that mediates type-2 immunity. Nature. 2010;464(7293):1367–70. doi:10.1038/nature08900.

114. Price AE, Liang HE, Sullivan BM, Reinhardt RL, Eisley CJ, Erle DJ, et al. Systemically dispersed innate IL-13-expressing cells in type 2 immunity. Proc Natl Acad Sci U S A. 2010;107(25):11489–94. doi:10.1073/pnas.1003988107.

115. Halim TY, Steer CA, Matha L, Gold MJ, Martinez-Gonzalez I, McNagny KM, et al. Group 2 innate lymphoid cells are critical for the initiation of adaptive T helper 2 cell-mediated allergic lung inflammation. Immunity. 2014;40(3):425–35. doi:10.1016/j.immuni.2014.01.011.

116. Halim TY, Hwang YY, Scanlon ST, Zaghouani H, Garbi N, Fallon PG, et al. Group 2 innate lymphoid cells license dendritic cells to potentiate memory Th2 cell responses. Nat Immunol. 2016;17(1):57–64. doi:10.1038/ni.3294.

117. Kemeny DM. The role of the T follicular helper cells in allergic disease. Cell Mol Immunol. 2012;9(5):386–9. doi:10.1038/cmi.2012.31.

118. Chtanova T, Tangye SG, Newton R, Frank N, Hodge MR, Rolph MS, et al. T follicular helper cells express a distinctive transcriptional profile, reflecting their role as non-Th1/Th2 effector cells that provide help for B cells. J Immunol. 2004;173(1):68–78.

119. Schaerli P, Willimann K, Lang AB, Lipp M, Loetscher P, Moser B. CXC chemokine receptor 5 expression defines follicular homing T cells with B cell helper function. J Exp Med. 2000;192(11):1553–62.

120. Walker LS, Gulbranson-Judge A, Flynn S, Brocker T, Raykundalia C, Goodall M, et al. Compromised OX40 function in CD28-deficient mice is linked with failure to develop CXC chemokine receptor 5-positive CD4 cells and germinal centers. J Exp Med. 1999;190(8):1115–22.

121. Kim CH, Rott LS, Clark-Lewis I, Campbell DJ, Wu L, Butcher EC. Subspecialization of CXCR5+ T cells: B helper activity is focused in a germinal center-localized subset of CXCR5+ T cells. J Exp Med. 2001;193(12):1373–81.

122. Butch AW, Chung GH, Hoffmann JW, Nahm MH. Cytokine expression by germinal center cells. J Immunol. 1993;150(1):39–47.

123. Vijayanand P, Seumois G, Simpson LJ, Abdul-Wajid S, Baumjohann D, Panduro M, et al. Interleukin-4 production by follicular helper T cells requires the conserved Il4 enhancer hypersensitivity site V. Immunity. 2012;36(2):175–87. doi:10.1016/j.immuni.2011.12.014.

124. Harada Y, Tanaka S, Motomura Y, Harada Y, Ohno S, Ohno S, et al. The 3′ enhancer CNS2 is a critical regulator of interleukin-4-mediated humoral immunity in follicular helper T cells. Immunity. 2012;36(2):188–200. doi:10.1016/j.immuni.2012.02.002.

Chapter 6
Traditional and Emerging Occupational Asthma in Japan

Kunio Dobashi

Abstract Occupational asthma (OA) is one of the most common forms of occupational lung disease in many industrialized countries, and it accounts for 9–15 % of adult asthma. If a worker with an occupational allergic disease doesn't consider it an occupational disease, or if affected workers bear it and take no measures or treatment, extensive exposure at the workplace will persist. These cause the disease to worsen or become refractory. Sometimes, patients might lose their job and face economic difficulties. Therefore, we should always take the possibility of OA into consideration and obtain a detailed history from patients. When OA is diagnosed, patients should avoid allergen exposure, and the workplace environment should be improved, as well as adequate drug therapy being provided. This paper covers the history, current state, and the published first guideline for diagnosis and management of occupational allergic diseases in Japan.

Keywords Occupational asthma • Konjac asthma • Guideline • Japan

6.1 History of OA in Japan

Occupational asthma (OA) is one of the most common forms of occupational lung disease in many industrialized countries, and it accounts for 9–15 % of adult asthma [1].

The first case of OA in Japan was reported in 1926 as "Asthma attack induced by working with American red cedar wood." When large amounts of American red cedar were imported for reconstruction after the Great Kanto Earthquake, carpenters suffered from asthma when processing this cedar. An epidemiological study revealed that approximately 10 % of carpenters were suffering from OA due to cedar. Therefore, import of the cedar was stopped and such OA was no longer seen.

K. Dobashi (✉)
Graduate School of Health Sciences, Gunma University,
3-39-22 Showa-machi, Maebashi, Gunma 371-8514, Japan
e-mail: dobashik@gunma-u.ac.jp

© Springer Science+Business Media Singapore 2017
T. Otsuki et al. (eds.), *Allergy and Immunotoxicology in Occupational Health*,
Current Topics in Environmental Health and Preventive Medicine,
DOI 10.1007/978-981-10-0351-6_6

After IgE was discovered in 1966, OA began to be studied from an immunological perspective. The first OA to be identified in Japan was konjac asthma. At that time, bronchial asthma apparently caused by "Maiko" powder was known among the residents living near konjac milling plants and the employees of these plants. A group from the First Department of Internal Medicine at Gunma University studied a detailed field survey in Shimonita that identified OA induced by inhaling Maiko powder, which they called konjac asthma and reported in 1951 [2]. After that, many OAs were reported as sea squirt asthma, silkworm phosphorus hair asthma, buckwheat asthma, silkworm cocoon asthma, and shiitake mushroom asthma in 1996, 1996, 1970, 1971, and 1985, respectively [3, 4].

6.2   Epidemiology of Occupational Asthma in Japan

The rate of the OAs is about 2–15 % of all asthmatics in Japan. However, we do not have correct data of incidence and prevalence of OA. Since it is possible that many patients are treated for asthma without diagnosis of OA, the actual prevalence is probably higher.

Among persons involved in specific types of work, the prevalence of OA depends on the allergens to which they are exposed or the work environment, and there are many reports about its prevalence (Table 6.1) [5, 6].

It is a serious problem that a high prevalence was shown around some factories because allergens released from the workplace cause residents living around the plants to develop asthma. We found that many residents living around a konjac factory had konjac asthma, and we proposed that this should be called "environmental asthma" (Table 6.2) [7].

Table 6.1 Estimated preverence of work-related asthma from cross-sectional studies in Japan

Type of work	Prevalence (%)
Konjac maker	5.0
Sericulturist	9.0
Polyurethane industry worker	16.4
Worker in plastic greenhouses of strawberry	4.6
Worker in plastic greenhouses of shiitake mushroom	5.0

Table 6.2 The number of Konjac asthma patients depend on the distance from the factories

Distance from factories	The number of Konjac asthma patients	The number of non-Konjac asthma patients
Within 300 m	46	17
300–1000 m	4	13
More than 1000 m	1	20

6.3 Allergens

The causative allergens are varied and sometimes unexpected. A part of substances that have been reported in Japan are summarized in Table 6.3 [7].

Causative allergens are divided into allergens of high molecular weight, such as those derived from animals and plants, and allergens of low molecular weight, such as chemicals and metals. According to the development of industry, the incidence of asthma induced by high molecular weight compounds is decreasing. On the other hand, asthma induced by low molecular weight substances is increasing and has become a serious problem, recently [5, 6]. The problems in OAs caused by chemicals are that the specific IgE antibody cannot be easily detected and diagnosis is difficult.

Table 6.3 Reported occupational allergens in Japan

		Allergen	Occupation	Year and author
Plants	Cereal	Amorphophallus konjac	Konjac maker	1951 Shichijo
		Buckwheat	Buckwheat miller. soba restaurant worker	1971 Nakamura
		Wheat flour	Baker. confectionary makers	1971 Jyo
		Barley flour	Miller	1991 Noda
	Wood particle	Western red cedar	Wood processing industry worker	1926 Seki
		Zelkova	Wood processing industry worker	1982 Katsuya
		Mulberry	Furniture making industry worker	1969 Nakamura
		White birch	Wood processing worker	1979 Takamoto
		Lauan	Wood processing worker	1968 Aoki
		Quince	Wood processing worker	1975 Takahashi
		Boxwood	Wood processing worker	1985 Tawara
	Others	Coffee beans powder	Manufacturing plant worker	1985 Shirakawa
		Sesame	Manufacturing plant worker sesame oil	1990 Tadokoro
		Tea leaf		
		Fresh top	Tea picking worker	1976 Ebihara
		Component of tea leaf	Tea manufacture worker	1989 Otsuka
		Tomato (component in stalk)	Worker in plastic greenhouses	1980 Saito
		Lettuce (component in stalk)	Worker in plastic greenhouses	1980 Saito
		Fuzz of melon	Worker in plastic greenhouses	1980 Masuyama

(continued)

Table 6.3 (continued)

		Allergen	Occupation	Year and author
Animal		Silk	Silk textile industry worker	1966 Nakamura
		Sea squirt	Oyster farm worker	1964 Jyo
		Alcyonarian	Japanese spiny lobster	1989 Onizuka
		Animal hair	Writing brush maker	1968 Kikuchi
		Mixed fertilizer (fish, crab)	Fertilizer factory worker	1982 Usami, 1991 Kasiwagi
		Sardine powder	Dried sardine factory worker	1987 Takamoto
		Coat of rat and guinea pig	Researcher	1972 Kobayashi
Pollen, spore	Pollen	Sugar beet	Researcher of sugar beet	1970 Matsuyama
		Rose	Researcher of rose	1978 Saito
		Orchard grass	Commercial grower of orchard grass	1971 Nakazawa
		Strawberry	Worker in plastic greenhouses of strawberry	1973 Kobayashi
		Peach	Commercial grower of peach	1973 shida
		Apple	Artificial pollination worker	1978 Sawada
		Grape	Worker in plastic greenhouses	1984 Tsukioka
		Pepper	Worker in plastic greenhouses	1985 Okumura
	Spore	Shiitake mushroom	Worker in plastic greenhouses	1968 Kondo
		Club moss	Dental technician	1969 Nakamura
		Smut fungus	Commercial grower of wheat.	1983 Asai
Metal, chemical	Drug	Diastase	Pharmacist; at drugstore;	1970 Fueki
		Pancreatin	Pharmacist; at drugstore;	1971 Nakamura
		Semisynthetic penicillin	Pharmacist; at drugstore;	1974 Kanetani
	Metal	Dichromate	Workers of cement producing industry	1972 Fueki
		Chloroplatinate	Industry worker	1984 Shima
	Chemical	TDI MDI	Polyurethane industry worker, painter	1970 Shima
		Ethylenediamine	Plastic processing worker	1979 Nakazawa
		Tetryl (explosive)	Pyrotechnist	1989 Inagaki
		Acrylic resin emulsion	Painter	1990 Nakamura

6.4 Traditional Occupational Asthma in Japan

6.4.1 Konjac Asthma

As I have described previously, the first OA to be identified immunologically in Japan was konjac asthma [2]. Konjac root is dried and ground into powder in the process of manufacturing the food known as konjac (no calorie food). Maiko is a fine konjac root powder that is blown by air pressure to obtain konjac powder for commercial use. Much of the Maiko powder is dispersed in the air and induces asthma in the plant workers by inhalation. The prevalence of konjac asthma was 16.6 % among employees in konjac mills, and the age of onset was different but mostly under 30 years.

The purified allergen of konjac asthma named Ag40D-2 is an acidic protein of about 24,000 daltons. Its ratio of basic to acidic amino acids is 1:3.7 and it induces a strong P-K reaction.

The immediate skin reaction to a purified Maiko powder allergen is positive in 100 % of konjac asthma patients, but negative in non-konjac asthma patients.

When the asthma was discovered, konjac making was an important industry in the Shimonita area and 40 % of the population were involved in producing konjac flour. Therefore, specific immunotherapy was developed because of the difficulty in changing jobs. When its efficacy was assessed, it was remarkably effective in 6/35 persons (17.1 %) and was effective in 18 (51.4 %) [3, 4].

After the konjac asthma was reported, companies began to improve the work environment. As a result of great effort, no one has developed konjac asthma since the late 1980s.

6.4.2 Sea Squirt Asthma

Sea squirt asthma is triggered by the inhalation of fluid from protochordate sea squirts that is adherent to cultured oysters. Cultivation of oysters in the Hiroshima region has been done for 400 years, and many people are engaged in the task of oyster husking. There were no reports before World War II, but employees complained of the onset of asthma associated with their work from around 1960. This asthma was reported in 1963 by Mitsui. In addition, detailed studies revealed that this type of asthma was induced by the inhalation of sea squirt components adherent to oysters. Such OA was named sea squirt asthma in 1966 [8].

The cause of its onset was improved farming methods that allowed farming of oysters in deep water since around 1952, so that sea squirts became attached to the oysters. Because work was often done under rough conditions with poor ventilation, workers inhaled a lot of sea squirt components.

From the investigation done at the time, the prevalence was 29 % (443 out of 1,528 people) and it reached 45.8 % in some towns. Because the industry has mostly female employees, there is a majority of female patients. Half of the patients develop asthma within 5 years of starting work.

Separation and purification of sea squirt allergen was carried out and four allergens (H, Gi-rep, Ei-M, and DIIIa) were identified. Especially Gi-rep and Ei-M were effective for immunotherapy.

The skin reaction to sea squirt allergen is positive in 91.3 % of sea squirt asthma patients. When an allergen inhalation challenge test was done with sea squirt allergen, four out of nine sea squirt asthma patients were positive.

Initially immunotherapy was done with the crude allergen and the efficacy rate was high at about 75 %. However, immunotherapy with the crude allergen caused side effects such as induction of asthma or urticaria. In contrast, therapy with the purified allergen has a higher efficacy rate of 91.5 % and causes fewer side effects [8].

As a result of great effort to improve work environments, the number of patients has recently shown a significant decrease due to improvement of the work environment.

6.5 Emerging Occupational Asthma

6.5.1 High Molecular Weight Allergen

The pollen of vegetables and fruits or spores of mushrooms have become causative allergens along with the increase of greenhouse culture. Especially, shiitake mushroom, tomato, and strawberry were not recognized as causing asthma when open-field cultivation was common.

Furthermore, it was reported that a furniture craftsman developed asthma by inhalation of the dust of *Albizia falcataria* (Falcata wood), which is a broad-leafed tree and began to be imported recently.

6.5.2 Low Molecular Allergen

There have been reports about occupational allergy induced by ortho-phthalaldehyde, which is used as a disinfectant solution for fiberscopes. Cases of ortho-phthalaldehyde-induced anaphylaxis began to be reported from around 2006. For example, anaphylaxis has occurred immediately after observation by a laryngeal fiberscope. Since various new chemicals will be developed in the future, we always have to pay attention to allergies caused by chemicals.

6.6 The First Guidelines for Occupational Allergic Diseases in Japan

6.6.1 Necessity of Guideline

It is extremely important to identify occupational allergic disease cases in their early stages and take appropriate preventive measures for the social lives of patients. A guideline was released in Canada as long ago as 1998, while the American Thoracic Society (ATS) guidelines were published in 2005 [1]. In the same year, other guidelines were published in the United Kingdom. Other guidelines that described diagnosis and management in detail were published by The American College of Chest Physicians, while more guidelines were released in Spain (in 2006) and in Singapore (in 2008). These guidelines show wide recognition of the importance of occupational asthma.

In Japan, a large number of case reports have been accumulated on occupational allergic diseases. However, because of the occupational features of the diseases, only case reports have been presented in many cases. Although guidelines for individual allergic diseases have been published by allergologic associations, the descriptions of occupational factors are generally minimal. It is extremely important that the guideline for diagnosis and management of occupational allergic diseases have been published in 2013 for the first time in Japan [5] (Fig. 6.1).

This guideline is designed to assist healthcare professionals engaging in ordinary diagnosis and management of allergic diseases to practice early detection and treatment and early prevention in patients with allergic diseases induced and worsened by occupational factors. We hope that this guideline will be used for ordinary diagnosis and management of occupational allergic diseases and help the patients.

6.6.2 The Structure of the Guideline

The guideline has a basic structure in which clinical questions are set with reference to Medical Information Network Distribution Service (MINDS); statements by the committee are listed; recommendation grades and evidence levels are defined; descriptions and references are indicated. Also, legal aspects are written in full.

As for occupational allergic diseases, because new substances have been continually produced due to technical innovation and working environments have been changing due to changes in industrial structures, new OAs can always arise. We have revised the guideline in 2016 and will continue to revise it every 3 years, in order to maintain a high level of evidence for the guideline.

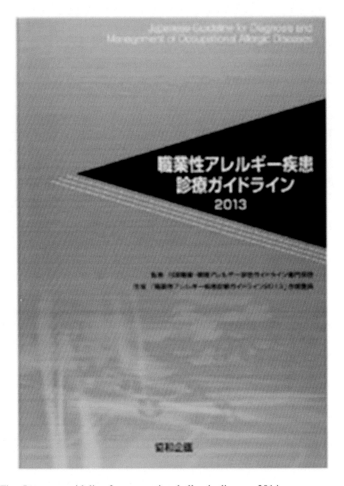

Fig. 6.1 First Japanese guideline for occupational allergic diseases 2014

6.7 Problems Related to Occupational Asthma in Japan

1. Due to advances in medication, achieving control of symptoms medically tends to be emphasized, and the search for causative allergens tends to be neglected. Thus, physicians often do not try to identify the causative allergen.
2. Poor surveillance data.
3. Poor regulation by law.
4. The work environment has improved in large enterprises under the direction of the government, but the smaller companies are not considered to have made enough effort in some cases.

6.8 Action Plans

1. Make surveillance system/checkup lung conditions of workers regularly.
2. Revise the guidelines of prevention and control of OA at stated periods.
3. OA information center and homepage are required.
4. Share information on OA in other countries.
5. Education about OA for workers, employers, healthcare providers, and government agencies.

References

1. Mapp CE, et al. Occupational asthma. Am J Respir Crit Care Med. 2005;172(3):280–305.
2. Shitijyo K. The study of Konnyaku asthma. Kitakannto Med J. 1951;1:29–30.
3. allergy, J.c.o.o, editor. Occupational asthma. Tokyo: Asakura Publishing Co., LTD; 1973.
4. allergy, J.c.o.o, editor. Occupational allergy. Tokyo: Buneido Publishing Co., LTD; 1983.
5. Committee for Japanese Guideline for Diagnosis and Management of Occupational Allergic Diseases. Japanese guideline for diagnosis and management of occupational allergic diseases 2013. Tokyo: Kyowa Kikaku; 2013 (in Japanese).
6. Dobashi K, et al. Japanese guideline for occupational allergic diseases 2014. Allergol Int. 2014;63(3):421–42.
7. Dobashi K. Occupational allergy. In: Fukuda T, editor. Sogo allergy-gaku. Tokyo: Nanzando; 2010.
8. Katsuya T. Hoya (Sea-Squirt) asthma (Japanese). Occup Environ Allergy. 2005;12:1–15.

Chapter 7
Skin Sensitization Model Based on Only Animal Data by Qualitative Structure-Toxicity Relationships (QSTR) Approach

Kazuhiro Sato, Kohtaro Yuta, and Yukinori Kusaka

Abstract Contact dermatitis is by far the most common form of occupational skin illness. *In silico* assessment of skin sensitization is increasingly needed owing to the problems concerning animal welfare, as well as excessive time consumed and cost involved in the development and testing of new chemicals.

We previously made skin sensitization model from human and animal data and reported. Its accuracy was 61.2 % (sensitivity 60.7 %, specificity 62.8 %) by external validation. This time we made skin sensitization QSTR model from only animal data (local lymph node assay (LLNA), 471 chemicals) by using K-step Yard sampling (KY) methods (US Patent No. 7725413, 2010) and 1 model KY method (US Patent Application).

A total of 320 compounds (212 positive sensitizers and 108 negative sensitizers) were used in this study. Two hundred and eighty-eight compounds were used to make a QSTR model and external validation study was performed by 32 compounds. The concordance of QSTR prediction for LLNA data was 71.9 % (sensitivity 54.5 %, specificity 81 %) and better than previous report. The concordance was better than previous time and indicates that the data of human and animal study were qualitatively different from each other.

Keywords Skin sensitization • Alternative methods • Qualitative structure-toxicity relationships (QSTRs) • Animal welfare

K. Sato (✉) • Y. Kusaka
Department of Environmental Health, School of Medicine, University of Fukui,
Fukui 910-1193, Japan
e-mail: satokazu@u-fukui.ac.jp

K. Yuta
In Silico Data Co Ltd, Narashino, Chiba 275-0025, Japan

© Springer Science+Business Media Singapore 2017
T. Otsuki et al. (eds.), *Allergy and Immunotoxicology in Occupational Health*,
Current Topics in Environmental Health and Preventive Medicine,
DOI 10.1007/978-981-10-0351-6_7

7.1 Introduction

In occupational health, occupational skin disorders are the most common. Among them, contact dermatitis is by far the most common form of occupational illness [1].

Under the new European Union (EU) Registration, Evaluation, and Authorization of Chemicals (REACH) rules, all chemicals in the EU that are produced or imported in quantities of more than 1 ton per annum need to be assessed as potential human and environmental hazards, for example, in terms of their carcinogenicity and human sensitivity, such chemicals also need to be determined. REACH calls for increased use of hazard assessment alternatives such as *in vitro* methods and QSTRs [2].

Since only two *in vitro* replacements are currently available for skin sensitization [3, 4], the use of QSTR approaches presents an attractive alternative [5]. One of the most difficult subjects in QSTR research is computer classification and prediction of chemical toxicity of compounds. This is because (1) there is large structural diversity among samples, (2) the sample number is enormously large, and (3) high classification and prediction rates are required. Nonlinear discriminant functions, such as neural network (NN), support vector machine (SVM), and AdaBoost, sometimes provide higher classification rate than that of linear methods. However, nonlinear methods are often accompanied by over-fitting which lowers prediction rate significantly.

Previously, we made the QSTR models for skin sensitization [6, 7], which are statistically based model [6], and the model by KY methods [7, 8] using animal-human mixed data based on human epidemiological studies, case reports, or validated animal studies (guinea pig maximization test, Buehler guinea pig test [9, 10]. The correct classification of our previous model by KY methods was 61.2 % (sensitivity 60.7 %, specificity 62.8 %). These KY methods can be applied to a linear and nonlinear discriminant function. The KY methods could classify a set of Ames test samples (6,965 compounds, 2,932 positive, 4033 negative) into two classes (positive/negative) correctly by 23 steps (data are not shown).

In this paper, we illustrate the KY methods, 1 model KY methods (US Patent Application), and only animal data (murine local lymph node assay) [11] based on our new model by KY methods and 1 model KY methods [7, 8].

7.2 Materials and Methods

7.2.1 Chemicals

Positive and negative 471 chemicals were obtained from the Interagency Coordinating Committee on the Validation of Alternative Methods (ICCVAM) Test Method Evaluation Report, the reduced murine local lymph node assay [11]. The criteria of positive data are more than three of stimulation index. However, inorganic chemicals, organic metal compounds, and polymers are special compounds and cannot be analyzed with general organic compounds in computational chemistry. Therefore, we deleted these chemicals and finally assessed 320 (212 positive and 108 negative) compounds. Two hundred and eighty-eight chemicals were used for learning set and 32 chemicals are used for external validation study (10 % cross-validation).

7.2.2   Parameters and Discriminant Functions

A total of 320 compounds (212 positive and 108 negative) were used for analysis. Two hundred and eighty-eight chemicals were used for learning set and 32 chemicals were used for 10 % cross-validation study (10 % CV). Parameters were generated from 2-D and 3-D structures of the compounds. The generated parameters were reduced by various feature selection (e.g., removing low appearance parameter, high correlation, or multicollinearity) methods. The KY methods were applied [7, 8]. In this case, AdaBoost and the iterative least squares linear discriminant functions (TILSQ) were used for generating discriminant functions.

7.2.3   KY Methods

Existing binary classifiers generate only one discriminant function in order to classify a sample set into two classes (Fig. 7.1). The same is true in the case of newly developed nonlinear classification methods, such as NN, SVM, and AdaBoost.

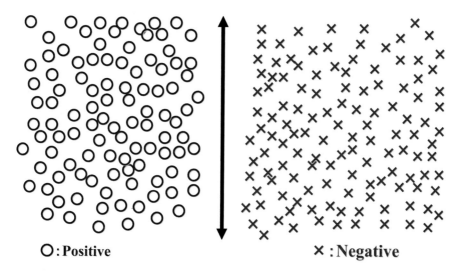

O : Positive   ✕ : Negative

Fig. 7.1 Linear discriminant function to classify all samples [7]

These nonlinear methods sometimes provide a higher classification rate than those of linear methods. However, if the samples highly overlapped one another, linear and nonlinear methods cannot classify the samples correctly into two classes (Fig. 7.2).

In the process of the KY methods, two different types of discriminant functions were created to determine positive, negative, and gray zones (Fig. 7.3). One of the discriminant functions is called as all-negative (AN) model and the other as all-positive (AP) model. The AN model classified AN samples in the sample set correctly and the AP model classified all-positive samples correctly. The samples which were classified as negative samples by AN model and positive samples by AP model belonged to the gray zone (Fig. 7.3).

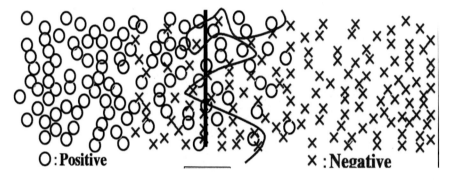

O : Positive _____ **× : Negative**

Fig. 7.2 Highly overlapped samples could not be classified completely by linear and nonlinear discriminant function [7]

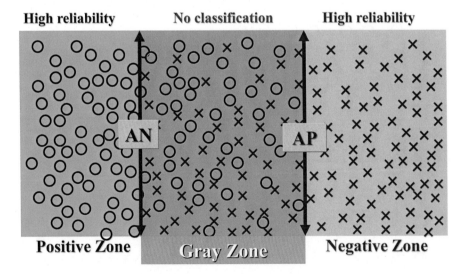

High reliability   **No classification**   **High reliability**

AN   **AP**

Positive Zone   **Gray Zone**   **Negative Zone**

Fig. 7.3 Classification results by AP and AN sample discriminant functions. Samples in positive zone and negative zone had high reliability of classification. *Gray* zone was not classified [7]

The KY methods focused on both sides of a sample space and found that there were special spaces, which included only correctly classified samples. These two areas have been defined as positive zone and the others as negative zone. The third zone was named as gray zone. All samples included in the positive zone belonged to a positive class, while all samples included in the negative zone belonged to a negative class. On the other hand, the samples included in the gray zone could not be determined whether they belonged to a positive or negative class since they were highly overlapped (Fig. 7.3).

If the gray zone (1) was determined by AN1 and AP1 discriminant functions, the gray zone (1) could be extracted and reclassified by AN2 and AP2 models to build a new sample set. If a new gray zone (2) was determined with respect to the new sample set, a further new sample set can be built as shown in Fig. 7.4. Repeating these steps, all samples in the original sample set can be classified correctly (Fig. 7.5). This is the basic concept of KY methods. The AN model and the AP model can be generated based on any conventional linear and nonlinear discriminant function. Therefore, KY methods can be categorized as a meta-algorithm approach.

All data analyses were performed using ADMEWORKS/Model Builder software (Fujitsu Kyushu Systems Limited, Japan).

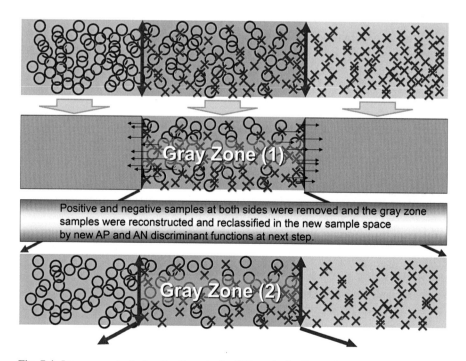

Fig. 7.4 Improvement of classification rate by KY methods. Correctly classified positive and negative samples are removed and the gray zone samples were reconstructed and reclassified in the new sample space by new discriminant functions at the next step [7]

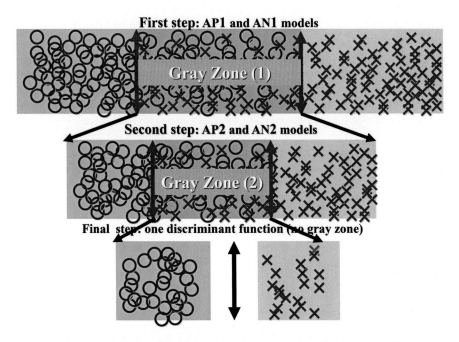

Fig. 7.5 Meta-algorithm repetition of reclassification of gray zone (KY methods). High reliability zone (correctly classified samples) was removed and gray zone was reclassified, and the sample space was reconstructed by new discriminant functions at the next step. All samples were correctly classified at the final step [7]

7.2.4   1 Model KY Methods

1 model KY methods are simple, easy, and delicately manipulated compared with ordinary 2 model KY methods (Fig. 7.6).

7.3   Results

In this study, AN and AP discriminant functions at step 1 were generated by AdaBoost. The final discriminant function was generated by TILSQ. All 288 compounds were perfectly classified by two steps.

The correct classification (10 % CV) of the KY methods was 71.9 % (sensitivity 54.5 %, specificity 81 %). That of 1 model KY methods was 69 %.

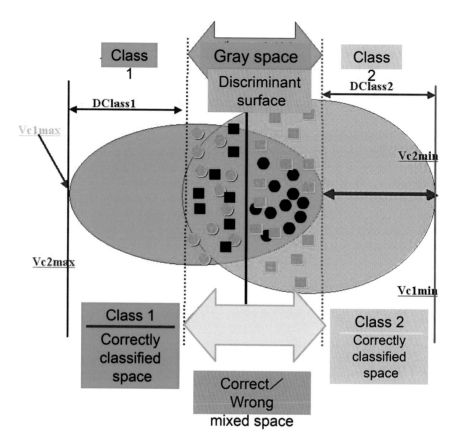

Fig. 7.6 1 model KY methods (overview)

7.4   Discussion

Since the implementation of Animal Welfare Guideline 86/09/EC in 1986, it is the declared policy of EU institutions to support the development and use of alternative methods of testing chemicals, that is, of "any method that can be used to reduce, replace or refine the use of animal experiments in biomedical research, testing or education" [12].

However, only two *in vitro* replacements are currently available for skin sensitization [3, 4]. Therefore, several QSTR-related systems have been developed for skin sensitization. These are Toxicity Prediction Komputer-Assisted Technology (Accelrys Inc., CA, USA; TOPKAT) and Multi-Computer Automated Structure Evaluation (MultiCASE Inc., Ohio, USA; M-CASE), which are both statistically based; Deductive Estimation of Risk from Existing Knowledge (DEREK) for Windows (DfW, LHASA Ltd., Leeds, UK), which is knowledge based; and Times

Metabolism Stimulator for Skin Sensitization (LMC, University of Bourgas, Bulgaria; TIMES-SS), which is a hybrid [13, 14].

In this study, the KY methods could be applied to this QSTR study. All 320 compounds were classified perfectly by a total of two steps. If only linear discriminant function is performed, these new methods always attain perfect classification rate without over-fitting, which causes lower prediction rate. This QSTR model applied AdaBoost and TILSQ. The correct classification rate of our previous QSTR model for skin sensitization by KY methods [7] was 62.5%. That of this model was 71.9% and better than that of previous study. These data indicated that the data of human and animal studies might be qualitatively different from each other. Guinea pig maximization test, Buehler test, and murine LLNA have only a 72–73% total accuracy of predicting actual human skin sensitizer [15, 16]. Our results might be appropriate. More research is needed to improve prediction rate.

We concluded that this QSTR system is thought to be applicable to initial prediction of skin sensitizing ability of untested chemicals and that the KY methods were promising tool in QSTR technology (classifying and predicting toxicity compounds).

Acknowledgments This work was supported by JSPS KAKENHI Grant Number 25293148.

References

1. Diepgen TL, Coenraads PI. 8. Occupational contact dermatitis. In: Rustermeyer T, Elsner P, John SM, Maibach HI, editors. Kanerva's occupational dermatology, vol. 1. Heidelberg: Springer; 2012. p. 51–83.
2. EU (2006) Regulation (EC) 1907/2006 of the European Parliament and the European Council of 18 December 2006 concerning the Registration, Evaluation, Authorization and Restriction of Chemicals (REACH), establishing a European Chemical Agency, amending Regulation 1999/45/EC and repeating Council Regulation (EEC) No 93/793 and Communication Regulation (EC) No 1488/94 as well as Council Directive 76/769/EEC and Commission Directive 91/155/EEC, 93/677/EEC and Commission Directive 91/155/EEC, 93/677/EEC, 93/105/EEC and 2000/21/EEC, Off J Eur Comm L vin P eds.
3. OECD (2015) Test guideline on an *In Chemico* Skin Sensitization: Direct Peptide Reactivity Assay (DPRA). OECD Guideline for the Testing of Chemicals No. 442C.
4. OECD (2015) Test guideline on an *in vitro* skin sensitization: ARE-Nrf2 luciferase test method. OECD guidelines for the testing of chemicals No. 442D..
5. Patlewicz G, Aptula AO, Roberts DW, Uriarte E. A minireview of available skin sensitization. (Q)SARs/expert systems. QSAR Comb Sci. 2008;27:60–76. doi:10.1002/qsar.200710067.
6. Sato K, Umemura T, Tamura T, Kusaka Y, et al. Skin sensitization study by quantitative structure-toxicity relationships (QSAR). AATEX. 2009;14:940–9. doi:10.11232/aatex.14.940.
7. Sato K, Umemura T, Tamura T, Kusaka Y, et al. Skin sensitization study by a new qualitative structure-toxicity relationships (QSTR) approach: K-step Yard Sampling (KY) methods. J Oral Tissue Eng. 2012;9(3):167–73. doi:10.11223/jarde.9.167doi.org/10.11223/jarde.9.167http.
8. K-step Yard sampling (KY) methods: Kohtaro Yuta, US Patent No: US7725413 B2 May 25, 2010.
9. Deutsche Forshungsgemeinshaft (DFG). IV. Sensitizing substances. In: List of MAK and BAT values. Alley-VCH, 2008. Weinheim, pp. 158–73.

10. Coz CJL, Lepoittevin JP. Dictionary of contact allergens: chemical sources, sources and references. In: Frosch PJ, Menne T, Lepoittevin JP, editors. Contact dermatitis. 4th ed. Berlin: Springer; 2006. p. 943–1105.
11. ICCVAM Test Method Evaluation Report. The reduced murine local lymph node assay: an alternative test method using fewer animals to assess the allergic contact dermatitis potential of chemicals and products. NIH Publication No. 09-6439. https://ntp.niehs.nih.gov/iccvam/docs/immunotox_docs/llna-ld/tmer.pdf. Accessed 15 Dec 2015.
12. Lilienblum W, Dekant W, Foth H, Gebel T, et al. Alternative methods to safety studies in experimental animals: role in the risk assessment of chemicals under the new European Chemicals Legislation (REACH). Arch Tocicol. 2008;82:211–36. doi:10.1007/s00204-008-0279-9.
13. Patlewicz G, Aptula AO, Uriarte E, Roberts DW, et al. An evaluation of selected global (Q) SARs/expert systems for the prediction of skin sensitization potential. SAR QSAR Environ Res. 2007;18:515–41. doi:10.1080/10629360701427872.
14. Patlewicz G, Dimitrov SD, Low LK, Kern PS, et al. TIMES-SS--a promising tool for the assessment of skin sensitization hazard. A characterization with respect to the OECD validation principles for (Q)SARs and an external evaluation for predictivity. Regul Toxicol Pharmacol. 2007;48:225–39. doi:10.1016/j.yrtph.2007.03.003.
15. Haneke KE, Tice RR, Carson BL, Margoin BH, Stokes WS. ICCVAM evaluation of the murine local lymph node assay. Data analyses completed by the National Toxicology Program Interagency Center for the Evaluation of Alternative Toxicological Methods. Regul Toxicol Pharmacol. 2001;34:274–86. doi:10.1006/rtph.2001.1498.
16. The murine local lymph node assay. The results of an independent peer review evaluation coordinated by the interagency coordinating committee on the validation of alternative methods (ICCVAM) and the National Toxicology Program Center for the Evaluation of Alternative Toxicological Methods (NICEATM). NIH publications no. 99-4494, 1999. Research Triangle Research.

Chapter 8
Non-industrial Indoor Environments and Work-Related Asthma

Nicola Murgia, Ilenia Folletti, Giulia Paolocci, Marco dell'Omo, and Giacomo Muzi

Abstract Work-related asthma is one of the most relevant work-related diseases worldwide, causing a high socio-economical burden. In the last decades, many countries experienced huge modifications in work organisations. These changes made people to move from traditional sectors to the tertiary sectors and non-industrial indoor working environments. Non-industrial indoor workplaces are characterised by a new concept of building, with a new structure, new materials, forced ventilation, tight construction and a potential exposure to new risk factors for work-related asthma, such as new chemicals and biological agents able to cause or exacerbate asthma. The actual scientific evidence suggests an increased risk of asthma among workers exposed to cleaning agents in indoor working environment and moulds in damp buildings. Also volatile organic compounds (VOCs) and environmental tobacco smoke could be considered triggers of asthma, even if their role is still under debate. Because of the increasing numbers of subjects working in non-industrial indoor environments and the scientific evidence of an increased risk of asthma in indoor environment, there is a need of public health intervention towards the prevention of work-related asthma, also in this specific setting.

Keywords Asthma • Indoor air • Moulds • Cleaning • Dampness

8.1 Introduction

Work-related asthma is one of the leading work-related diseases worldwide; 15 % of all cases of asthma are related to workplace exposures [1]. Current guidelines and statements divide work-related asthma in occupational asthma, directly caused by a specific exposure at the workplace, and work-exacerbated asthma, a form of common asthma which is aggravated by occupational exposure [2]. Many occupational

N. Murgia (✉) • I. Folletti • G. Paolocci • M. dell'Omo • G. Muzi
Section of Occupational Medicine, Respiratory Diseases and Toxicology, University of Perugia, Piazzale Severi 1, 06100 Perugia, Italy
e-mail: nicola.murgia@unipg.it

© Springer Science+Business Media Singapore 2017
T. Otsuki et al. (eds.), *Allergy and Immunotoxicology in Occupational Health*,
Current Topics in Environmental Health and Preventive Medicine,
DOI 10.1007/978-981-10-0351-6_8

exposures, around 250, have been found to cause directly or to exacerbate asthma. Chemicals causing or exacerbating asthma are usually divided into high molecular weight (HMW) agents (e.g. flour, animal allergens, latex, etc.), low molecular weight (LMW) agents (e.g. isocyanates, acrylates, etc.) and irritants. HMW and LMW show often an immunologic mechanism of action which is IgE mediated (HMW) or through a non-IgE Th2 response (LMW), while irritants are not showing a specific immunologic pattern, but sometimes an unspecific activation of the humoral response [2, 3].

These exposures may occur in many workplaces, both industrial and non-industrial. One important working environment, where exposure to asthmogenic substances may happen, is the non-industrial indoor workplaces.

8.2   Non-industrial Indoor Environment

The non-industrial indoor setting is a composite life and work environment used for housing (private houses, hotels, etc.), common social and health structures (hospitals, schools, etc.), leisure activities (bars, cinemas, sport halls), transportation (buses, trains, boats, etc.) and work (offices, hospitals, etc.). Nowadays, in North America, Europe and Japan, people are spending 80–90 % of their life in an indoor environment [4] and in their houses but also at work.

Modern indoor workplaces are very different from the past for their external and internal structure. They are usually placed in suburban areas and constituted by an internal load-bearing core and an external light frame. This structure allows to reach a considerable height, which is useful to reduce the land cost. Anyway, this kind of structure needs some adjustment to guarantee comfort and to reduce costs related to heating and cooling of the indoor environment. In new non-industrial indoor environments, measures essential to ensure comfort and reduce the costs are:

- Massive use of insulating material, which was asbestos in the past decades and now is man-made mineral or ceramic fibres
- Artificial ventilation, usually controlled remotely, which implies also the presence of "tight" buildings, to assure control and reduce the dispersion of heating or cooling
- Artificial lighting

Besides, in modern non-industrial indoor environments, for design and economical reason, interiors have been changed a lot during the last decades. Furnitures are now made mainly with light, low-cost, composite materials and resins, such as plywood, chipboard and urea-formaldehyde resins. Floors and walls are covered by plastic carpets. Computers and printers are the main working tools encountered in these workplaces. Finally, to ensure cleanness and hygiene, a wide range of chemical cleaning agents are used, particularly in indoor spaces dedicated to special purposes (e.g. hospitals and schools).

This indoor structure has also a great impact on work organisation and, despite obvious differences between countries in terms of materials, architecture and needs, is revolutionising the concept of work as human beings have thoughts in the previous centuries [5].

8.3 Indoor Air Pollutants

The new way of projecting and constructing new living and working settings, with the use of many new chemicals to build and keep clean the structure, has influenced greatly the indoor air quality. The American Society of Heating, Refrigerating and Air-conditioning Engineers, in its 2010 standard, defines indoor air as "acceptable" when known toxic chemicals are not present or below noxious concentrations and when the majority (>80%) of people living or working in that environment is not reporting symptoms or diseases. Non-industrial indoor air could contain many chemicals as VOCs, ozone, particulate matter, asbestos and man-made fibres and environmental tobacco smoke. Moreover, indoor air could be contaminated by biological (moulds, mites, bacteria and viruses) and physical (radon) hazards [6].

The source of indoor air pollution is mainly outdoor air but also building and furniture material release, human activity in the indoor environment, cleaning agents and poor maintenance of heating and ventilation system.

8.3.1 Physical Pollutants

8.3.1.1 Temperature, Ventilation and Humidity

Indoor environment temperature is one of the most important parameters influencing workers' health and productivity. High temperature and low humidity have been associated with respiratory and cutaneous symptoms, such as airway, eye and skin dryness, but also with more general symptoms (headache). As a matter of fact, low humidity and high ventilation have been associated with a quicker evaporation of the lacrimal film in indoor workers [7]. On the contrary, a too high humidity seems to increase discomfort in indoor working environments because of an increased release of bad smell from materials contaminated by moulds. In fact high humidity could increase the growth of fungi and dust mites, which could affect the health and wellness of workers staying indoor [8]. Nevertheless, temperature and humidity could influence also the concentration of chemicals in indoor air, especially particulate matter and chemicals released by furniture, insulation material and carpets. This would make difficult to understand whether symptoms related to indoor air are associated more with physical pollutants or with the influence of physical parameters on chemical composition of indoor air.

8.3.1.2 Radon

Radon is a natural radioactive carcinogenic compound, which is usually found in indoor air. It derives from the natural release from the soil where the building is placed. Radon high-releasing soils are volcanic rocks and materials (tuff, pozzolan, etc.) and granites. Radon is usually concentrated in lower floors, especially those underground, and its contamination is fostered by the natural flow between outside cold air and inside warmer air (the so-called chimney effect); ventilation is also an important factor which usually reduces the concentration of radon in indoor tight environments. Radon is a known carcinogenic compound for the International Agency for the Research on Cancer (IARC), and many studies have issued the problem of indoor air contamination in occupational and nonoccupational settings [9].

8.3.2 Chemical Pollutants

8.3.2.1 Formaldehyde

Formaldehyde is found in building materials and furniture (panels, plywood, chipboard, medium-density fibreboard (MDF)), glues, insulating foams, resins and environmental tobacco smoke. Formaldehyde in indoor air could come also from the reaction between ozone and other VOCs or aliphatic hydrocarbon (from printers) or alkanes (from cleaning products and air fresheners) [10]. The amount of formaldehyde released in the environments is higher for newly constructed living and working environments, including newly produced furniture. Moreover, formaldehyde concentration is influenced by temperature and humidity of indoor air. In offices formaldehyde concentration is around 0.045 mg/m^3; for these concentrations some worker could start to perceive formaldehyde smell as well to report various symptoms such as nose, throat, eyes and skin irritation, headache, sleepiness and dizziness [11]. Some studies highlighted a possible role of formaldehyde in causing asthma and rhinitis, by the interaction with other chemicals (ozone, VOCs) and directly enhancing the expression of adhesion molecules on nasal mucosa [12].The IARC has classified formaldehyde carcinogenic for human beings, because of its role in causing nasal cancer and other malignancies [13].

8.3.2.2 VOCs

VOCs are organic compounds found in indoor air, with a boiling point between 50 and 250 °C. They are rather many comprise of aliphatic and aromatic hydrocarbons, cycloalkanes, aldehydes, terpenes, alcohols, esters and ketones [14]. Major sources of VOCs are building materials, paints, glues, furnitures, cleaning products, printers and photocopiers. VOCs are also produced by chemical reaction between other chemicals, especially ozone and nitrous compounds, and by moulds (the so-called

MVOCs), being responsible of the bad smell often perceived in indoor environments. Exposure to VOCs has been associated with airway irritation, inflammation and obstruction and general symptoms (sleepiness, dizziness), even if this finding has not been always confirmed [15].

8.3.2.3 Ozone

Ozone concentration in indoor air is related to ozone in outdoor air, to ventilation, to reaction with other chemicals (ozone-initiated indoor chemistry) and to the release from furniture and building materials. Chemicals usually reacting with ozone in indoor environments are isoprene, styrene, terpenes, squalene and saturated and unsaturated fatty acids from furniture, carpets, cleaning products and air fresheners. One important source of ozone pollution in indoor air is the release by laser printers, photocopiers, electrostatic filters and precipitators [16].

Exposure to mild concentration of ozone (160 μg/m3) can cause airway irritation, inflammation, obstruction and bronchial hyperresponsiveness. Respiratory symptoms associated with ozone exposure are more frequent in subjects with pre-existent respiratory diseases. In allergic patients ozone could prime the airways enhancing the response to inhaled allergens. Genetic could explain the large variety of short-term reactions to ozone in different subjects. An increase in outdoor ozone concentration has been associated with an increased mortality and hospital admission for respiratory diseases. It has been also shown that outdoor exposure to ozone is correlated with higher morbidity for cardiovascular diseases [17].

8.3.2.4 Phthalates

Phthalates are a large family of chemical compounds used in the indoor environment to increase the flexibility and elasticity of polyvinylchloride-based carpets. Even if phthalates are mainly introduced in the body by the oral route, respiratory exposure by indoor air has been demonstrated. Phthalates are mainly known as endocrine disruptor, but some study pointed out a possible role in allergy and asthma [18].

8.3.2.5 Particulate Matter

Particulate matter (PM) is often classified by its diameter in ultrafine (PM 0.1), with a diameter <0.1 μm; in fine (PM 2.5), with a diameter <2.5 μm; and finally in PM10, with particles <10 μm. Fine particles are mainly produced during combustion and larger particles (PM10) are usually the results of fine-particle aggregation [19]. Major sources of particulate matter in indoor air are combustion process, tobacco smoke, laser printers and photocopiers [15]. Other less prominent sources are pollens, moulds, bacteria and sprays. Usually larger particles are coming mainly from outdoor through windows and the ventilation system. Toxic effects of particulate matter are related to its diameter, and larger particles affect the nose, throat and larger airways, while smaller particles, belonging to the respirable fraction, could directly affect small airways and alveoli. Moreover, the toxicity is also mediated by the substances (e.g. aromatic hydrocarbons, nitrous compounds, aldehydes) absorbed onto the particles' surface [20]. A large number of studies show that PM could be a strong eye and airway irritant and could exacerbate asthma. Nevertheless, some reports suggested a possible role of particulate matter to induce a direct alveoli inflammation with diffusing capacity impairment [15]. Long-term exposure to PM is able to increase morbidity and mortality for respiratory and cardiovascular disorders. Indoor air threshold for PM has not been established yet as it was done for outdoor exposure to PM.

8.3.2.6   Environmental Tobacco Smoke (ETS)

Exposure to environmental tobacco smoke (also named "passive smoking" or "second-hand tobacco smoke") is the inhalation of tobacco smoke by non-smoking subjects because of the presence of smokers in their same environment. ETS is one of the most import pollutants of indoor working environment [21]. Tobacco smoke accounts for more than 4000 toxic substances with carcinogenic, toxic and inflammatory effects. Health effects of tobacco smoke on airways are irritation and inflammation, causing asthma and chronic bronchitis exacerbations and increased susceptibility to respiratory infections. Long-term exposure is correlated with airway impairment and chronic obstructive pulmonary disease. ETS has been classified carcinogenic by the IARC, increasing the risk of lung cancer by 16–19% in occupational settings. Some reports suggest an increased risk also for breast cancer [22]. Recent smoking bans in different countries have reduced a lot the exposure to ETS. In indoor environment it has been described also the third-hand smoke phenomenon, when after ETS cessation, smoke-related chemicals can persist in the indoor environment absorbed onto the PM [23].

8.3.3   Biological Pollutants

In North America building dampness and the consequent mould overgrowth are considered the principal cause of indoor-related symptoms. Mould overgrowth is also related to ventilation and dehumidification system impairment [24]. The most important fungal species related to indoor pollutions are *Aspergillus versicolor*, *Penicillium brevicompactum*, *Penicillium chrysogenum* and *Cladosporium* species. Moulds can produce a biological effect by their capacity to elicit an immune response, causing rhinitis, asthma and even more dangerous diseases, such as hypersensitivity pneumonitis and allergic bronchopulmonary aspergillosis. Besides, moulds could cause a direct irritating effect on the eyes, airways and skin [25]. Dust mite is another important biological indoor pollutant capable of causing sensitisation and consequently rhinitis, dermatitis and asthma. In the European Community Respiratory Health Survey, indoor contamination by dust mites has been extensively studied, finding differences in dust mites' contamination across countries, depending mainly on the indoor humidity [26].

8.4   Asthma and Non-industrial Indoor Workplaces

The relation between asthma and exposure to occupational indoor pollutants has been extensively studied in the last decades in North America, Europe and Asia because of the socio-economical changes, which moved people from farming and industry to the tertiary sector.

Occupational exposures to cleaning agents, disinfectants and moulds are the fields more frequently studied, even if also other exposures have been associated with the onset or the exacerbation of asthma.

8.4.1   Exposure to Cleaning Agents and Disinfectant: The Health-Care Sector

Cleaning agents are mostly irritants for the airways and thus they could act as other factors associated with work-related irritant asthma. Glutaraldehyde, a typical disinfectant used in hospitals to clean endoscopes, has shown also the capacity to cause an immunologic reaction through an IgE-mediated mechanism. Studies performed on health-care personnel and professional cleaners working in hospital have shown an increased risk of work-related asthma due to the exposure to traditional cleaning agents (bleach, ammonia, detergents), especially if cleaning agents and disinfectants are used in their sprayed form [27]. There is also a moderate scientific evidence that exposure to specific disinfectant agents for health-care settings (glutaraldehyde, formaldehyde, ethylene oxide) is correlated with work-related asthma and work-related respiratory symptoms [28]. In Asia and Europe, nurses have shown an increased risk of hospitalisation for asthma and new-onset asthma, especially if exposed to cleaning agents [29, 30].

In hospital technician the use of ammonia or bleach as cleaning agents has been associated with an increased risk of respiratory symptoms [31].

8.4.2   Exposure to Cleaning Agents and Disinfectant: Other Sectors

As in the health-care sector in other sectors, cleaning agents have mainly an irritating effect. In professional cleaners the exposure to detergents seems to increase the risk of respiratory symptoms and asthma, with an effect related also to the exposure duration and the use of sprayed cleaning agents [32, 33]. In larger studies the association between professional cleaning and respiratory symptoms was rather clear, while an effect on asthma occurrence was not evident. The tasks showing a correlation with respiratory symptoms are dewaxing, carpet and wall cleaning [34]. In other studies, exposure to ammonia was able to exacerbate a pre-existent asthma [35]. Finally, long-term exposure to cleaning agents was associated with an accelerated FEV1 decline in professional cleaners [31].

8.4.3 Exposure to Moulds

Mould exposure at work can cause allergic sensitisation and consequently a typical allergic asthma due to fungal spores. As it is written above, exposure to *Aspergillus* spp. could cause a rare form of sensitisation, the allergic bronchopulmonary aspergillosis, a severe disease resembling asthma in some of the first stages, but more difficult to treat. In some case moulds can cause the production of irritating compounds, such as aldehydes or particulate, which may act on the airway directly, without a cellular immunologic response. Workplace dampness and the consequent mould overgrowth are relevant public health problems in many countries. Office and school dampness increases the prevalence of asthma and wheezing among, respectively, clerks and teachers [36, 37]. Dampness was able to increase sickness absence due to asthma in clerks [38]. Mould exposure at the workplace was also associated with increased bronchial hyperresponsiveness [39]. Workplace dampness has been found to increase the concentration of exhaled breath inflammatory biomarkers [40]. The association between visible moulds at the workplace and asthma is consistent also with the duration of exposure; as a matter of fact the effect was stronger when a visible damage was present at the workplace for more than 5 years [41]. Environmental assessment of fungal growth was associated with asthma onset [42].

8.4.4 Other Exposures

Indoor swimming pool workers have been found at higher risk of asthma because of the exposure to disinfectants (trihalomethane, trichloramine), with a dose-response relationship [43, 44]. In this case the effect of these substances is irritating and usually can be resolved reducing the concentration of chemicals used to sanitise water [45].

Workers exposed to ETS in indoor non-industrial working environments seem to be at higher risk of asthma symptoms [46], in this case the role of passive smoking is not completely clear, and it could act as a mixture of irritating compounds but also enhance the sensitisation to indoor allergen, as it is happening in children exposed to ETS. More debated is the role of occupational exposure to nitrogen oxides occurring in ice sport arenas or kitchen and the occurrence of work-related asthma; in this case the mechanism is largely unknown, even if in hockey players, a mixed neutro-philic and eosinophilic inflammation was found analysing induced sputum, after the training [47, 48]. Less evidence is provided about the role of ozone and particulate released by laser printers and photocopiers on asthma onset [49, 50].

8.5   Conclusions

Economy, technology and work organisation have changed workplaces enormously in the last 30 years. Besides, the number of workers involved in the tertiary sector is constantly rising. These factors increased the attention to this new working environment, previously considered safe.

There is a scientific evidence that the occupational exposure to cleaning agents and disinfectant occurring in non-industrial indoor settings are associated with asthma onset or exacerbation. Moreover, exposure to moulds in damp building, especially in North America and Northern Europe, plays an important role in determining or exacerbating asthma. The role of other indoor occupational exposures, especially ETS, is not completely clear but could contribute to the burden of work-related asthma. In conclusion, because of the high socio-economical burden of work-related asthma and the increasing number of subjects working in non-industrial indoor environment, there is an urgent need of public health intervention to avoid or reduce the exposure to risk factors associated with indoor air-related asthma. The intervention must start during the design and planning phase of new buildings, to prevent the release of toxic substance from building materials and furniture, as well as to reduce the risk of mould contamination. Afterwards, attention must be paid to the use of non-toxic cleaning agents and to keep the ventilation system working properly. Workers' health surveillance could play an important role in primary and, overall, in secondary prevention. Information of workers, especially those involved in professional cleaning, is very important to discourage dangerous habits, such as mixing reactive and irritant chemicals, and to implement the use of personal protective equipment, when appropriate.

References

1. Lemiere C. Occupational and work-exacerbated asthma: similarities and differences. Expert Rev Respir Med. 2007;1(1):43–9.
2. Tarlo SM, Balmes J, Balkissoon R, Beach J, Beckett W, Bernstein D, Blanc PD, Brooks SM, Cowl CT, Daroowalla F, Harber P, Lemiere C, Liss GM, Pacheco KA, Redlich CA, Rowe B, Heitzer J. Diagnosis and management of work-related asthma: American College of Chest Physicians Consensus Statement. Chest. 2008;134(3 Suppl):1S–41.
3. Bernstein DI. Occupational asthma caused by exposure to low-molecular-weight chemicals. Immunol Allergy Clin North Am. 2003;23(2):221–34.

4. Leech JA, Nelson WC, Burnett RT, et al. It's about time: a comparison of Canadian and American time-activity patterns. J Expo Anal Environ Epidemiol. 2002;12:427–32.
5. Muzi G, dell'Omo M, Murgia N, Abbritti G. Chemical pollution of indoor air and its effects on health. G Ital Med Lav Ergon. 2004;26(4):364–9.
6. ASHRAE, ANSI/ASHRAE Standard 62.1-2010. Ventilation for acceptable indoor air quality. Atlanta: American Society of Heating, Refrigerating, and Air-Conditioning Engineers, Inc; 2010.
7. Wolkoff P. "Healthy" eye in office-like environments. Environ Int. 2008;34(8):1204–14.
8. Mendell MJ, Mirer AG, Cheung K, Tong M, Douwes J. Respiratory and allergic health effects of dampness, mold, and dampness-related agents: a review of the epidemiologic evidence. Environ Health Perspect. 2011;119:748–56.
9. WHO guidelines for indoor air quality: selected pollutants. Geneva: World Health Organization; 2010.
10. Wolkoff P, Nielsen GD. Non-cancer effects of formaldehyde and relevance for setting an indoor air guideline. Environ Int. 2010;36:788–99.
11. Paustenbach D, Alarie Y, Kulle T, et al. A recommended occupational exposure limit for formaldehyde based on irritation. J Toxicol Environ Health. 1997;50(3):217–63.
12. Kim WJ, Terada N, Nomura T, Takahashi R, Lee SD, Park JH, Konno A. Effects of formaldehyde on the expression of adhesion molecules in nasal microvascular endothelial cells: the role of formaldehyde in the pathogenesis of sick building syndrome. Clin Exp Allergy. 2002;32:287–95.
13. Nielsen GD, Wolkoff P. Cancer effects of formaldehyde: a proposal for an indoor air guideline value. Arch Toxicol. 2010;84:423–46.
14. Hodgson AT, Bea J, McIlvaine JE. Sources of formaldehyde, other aldehydes and terpenes in a new manufactured house. Indoor Air. 2002;12:235–42.
15. Wolkoff P. Indoor air pollutants in office environments: assessment of comfort, health, and performance. Int J Hyg Environ Health. 2012;216:371–94.
16. Weschler CJ. Ozone's impact on public health: contributions from indoor exposures to ozone and products of ozone-initiated chemistry. Environ Health Perspect. 2006;114(10):1489–96.
17. Devlin RB, Duncan KE, Jardim M, Schmitt MT, Rappold AG, Diaz-Sanchez D. Controlled exposure of healthy young volunteers to ozone causes cardiovascular effects. Circulation. 2012;126:104–11.
18. North ML, Takaro TK, Diamond ML, Ellis AK. Effects of phthalates on the development and expression of allergic disease and asthma. Ann Allergy Asthma Immunol. 2014;112(6):496–502.
19. Hulin M, Simoni M, Viegi G, Annesi-Maesano I. Respiratory health and indoor air pollutants based on quantitative exposure assessments. Eur Respir J. 2012;40:1033–45.
20. Bernstein JA, Alexis N, Bacchus H, et al. The health effects of non-industrial indoor air pollution. J Allergy Clin Immunol. 2008;121:585–91.
21. US Surgeon General. Passive smoke. The health consequences of involuntary exposure to tobacco smoke: a report of the Surgeon General. Office on Smoking and Health (US). Atlanta: Centers for Disease Control and Prevention (US); 2006.
22. Jaakkola MS, Jaakkola JJK. Assessment of exposure to environmental tobacco smoke. Eur Respir J. 1997;10:2384–97.
23. Kuschner WG, Reddy S, Mehrotra N, Paintal HS. Electronic cigarettes and thirdhand tobacco smoke: two emerging health care challenges for the primary care provider. Int J Genet Med. 2011;4:115–20.
24. ASHRAE. Indoor air quality guide: best practices for design, construction and commissioning. Atlanta: ASHRAE; 2009. p. 24–50.
25. Fisk WJ, Lei-Gomez Q, Mendell MJ. Meta-analyses of the associations of respiratory health effects with dampness and molds in homes. Indoor Air. 2007;17(4):284–96.

26. Zock JP, Heinrich J, Jarvis D, Verlato G, Norback D, Plana E, Sunyer J, Chinn S, Olivieri M. Distribution and determinants of house dust mite allergens in Europe: the European Community Respiratory Health Survey II. Allergy Clin Immunol. 2006;118:682–90.
27. Dumas O, Donnay C, Heederik DJ, Héry M, Choudat D, Kauffmann F, Le Moual N. Occupational exposure to cleaning products and asthma in hospital workers. Occup Environ Med. 2012;69(12):883–9.
28. Arif AA, Delclos GL. Association between cleaning-related chemicals and work-related asthma and asthma symptoms among healthcare professionals. Occup Environ Med. 2012;69(1):35–40.
29. Li X, Sundquist J, Sundquist K. Socioeconomic and occupational groups and risk of asthma in Sweden. Occup Med (London). 2008;58(3):161–8.
30. Kogevinas M, Zock JP, et al. Exposure to substances in the workplace and new-onset asthma: an international prospective population-based study (ECRHS-II). Lancet. 2007;370(9584):336–41.
31. Mirabelli MC, London SJ, Charles LE, Pompeii LA, Wagenknecht LE. Occupation and three-year incidence of respiratory symptoms and lung function decline: the ARIC Study. Respir Res. 2012;13:24. doi:10.1186/1465-9921-13-24.
32. De Fátima Maçãira E, Algranti E, Medina Coeli Mendonça E, Antônio Bussacos M. Rhinitis and asthma symptoms in non-domestic cleaners from the Sao Paulo metropolitan area, Brazil. Occup Environ Med. 2007;64(7):446–53.
33. Orriols R, Costa R, Albanell M, Alberti C, Castejon J, Monso E, Panades R, Rubira N, Rubira N, Zock JP, Malaltia Ocupacional Respiratória (MOR) Group. Reported occupational respiratory diseases in Catalonia. Occup Environ Med. 2006;63(4):255–60.
34. Obadia M, Liss GM, Lou W, Purdham J, Tarlo SM. Relationships between asthma and work exposures among non-domestic cleaners in Ontario. Am J Ind Med. 2009;52(9):716–23.
35. Lemiere C, Bégin D, Camus M, Forget A, Boulet LP, Gérin M. Occupational risk factors associated with work-exacerbated asthma in Quebec. Occup Environ Med. 2012;69(12):901–7.
36. Laney AS, Cragin LA, et al. Sarcoidosis, asthma, and asthma-like symptoms among occupants of a historically water-damaged office building. Indoor Air. 2009;19(1):83–90.
37. Sahakian N, Park JH, Cox-Ganser J. Respiratory morbidity and medical visits associated with dampness and air-conditioning in offices and homes. Indoor Air. 2009;19(1):58–67.
38. Sahakian NM, White SK, Park JH, Cox-Ganser JM, Kreiss K. Identification of mold and dampness-associated respiratory morbidity in 2 schools: comparison of questionnaire survey responses to national data. J Sch Health. 2008;78(1):32–7.
39. Karvala K, Toskala E, Karvala K, Toskala E, Luukkonen R, Uitti J, Lappalainen S, Nordman H. Prolonged exposure to damp and moldy workplaces and new-onset asthma. Int Arch Occup Environ Health. 2011;84(7):713–21.
40. Akpinar-Elci M, Siegel PD, Cox-Ganser JM, Stemple KJ, White SK, Hilsbos K, Weissman DN. Respiratory inflammatory responses among occupants of a water-damaged office building. Indoor Air. 2008;18(2):125–30.
41. Karvala K, Toskala E, Luukkonen R, Lappalainen S, Uitti J, Nordman H. New-onset adult asthma in relation to damp and moldy workplaces. Int Arch Occup Environ Health. 2010;83(8):855–65.
42. Park JH, Cox-Ganser JM, Kreiss K, White SK, Rao CY. Hydrophilic fungi and ergosterol associated with respiratory illness in a water-damaged building. Environ Health Perspect. 2008;116(1):45–50.
43. Fantuzzi G, Predieri G, Giacobazzi P, Mastroianni K, Aggazzotti G. Prevalence of ocular, respiratory and cutaneous symptoms in indoor swimming pool workers and exposure to disinfection by-products (DBPs). Int J Environ Res Public Health. 2010;7(4):1379–91.
44. Jacobs JH, Spaan S, van Rooy GB, Meliefste C, Zaat VA, Rooyackers JM, Heederik D. Exposure to trichloramine and respiratory symptoms in indoor swimming pool workers. Eur Respir J. 2007;29(4):690–8.

45. Seys SF, Feyen L, Keirsbilck S, Adams E, Dupont LJ, Nemery B. An outbreak of swimming-pool related respiratory symptoms: an elusive source of trichloramine in a municipal indoor swimming pool. Int J Hyg Environ Health. 2015;218(4):386–91.
46. Eisner MD, Yelin EH, Katz PP, Earnest G, Blanc PD. Exposure to indoor combustion and adult asthma outcomes: environmental tobacco smoke, gas stoves, and woodsmoke. Thorax. 2002;57(11):973–8.
47. Lumme A, Haahtela T, Ounap J, Rytilä P, Obase Y, Helenius M, Remes V, Helenius I. Airway inflammation, bronchial hyperresponsiveness and asthma in elite ice hockey players. Eur Respir J. 2003;22(1):113–7.
48. Wong TW, Wong AH, Lee FS, Qiu H. Respiratory health and lung function in Chinese restaurant kitchen workers. Occup Environ Med. 2011;68(10):746–52.
49. Jaakkola MS, Jaakkola JJ. Office work exposures and adult-onset asthma. Environ Health Perspect. 2007;115(7):1007–11.
50. Yang CY, Haung YC. A cross sectional study of respiratory and irritant health symptoms in photocopier workers in Taiwan. J Toxicol Environ Health A. 2008;71(19):1314–7.

Chapter 9
Combined Effect on Immune and Nervous System of Aluminum Nanoparticles

Qiao Niu and Qinli Zhang

Abstract Aluminum is believed to be a neurotoxicant for a lot of years and thought to be related with Alzheimer's disease. In recent decades, aluminum nanoparticles have been utilized widely in many fields, and their potential adverse effect on health drew great concern. Al_2O_3 nanoparticles (ANPs) can be inhaled more deeply into the respiratory system, and translocated into the bloodstream to induce immunotoxicity and into the central nervous system to induce neurotoxicity, of which the possible mechanisms are summarized in this chapter. ANPs may induce pneumocyte apoptosis by triggering oxidative stress and inhibit or activate activity of cytokines, and the immunotoxicity induced by nanoalumina (Nano-Al) particles was higher than that of macro-sized alumina particles. Besides though blood compartment by which ANPs damage the blood-brain barrier, ANPs may enter into the central nervous system through the olfactory nerve. ANPs impair behavioral performance of model organisms and rodents. ANPs may induce neural cell death by triggering apoptosis, necrosis, and autophagy, complicate cell signal transmission pathways, and promote Aβ deposit and degeneration.

Keywords Alumina nanoparticle • Immunotoxicity • Oxidative stress • Neurotoxicity • Cell death • Signal pathway

Q. Niu (✉)
Occupational Health Department, Public Health School, Shanxi Medical University, Shanxy, Taiyuan 030001, China
e-mail: niuqiao55@163.com

Q. Zhang
Shanxi medical University, Taiyuan 030001, China

© Springer Science+Business Media Singapore 2017
T. Otsuki et al. (eds.), *Allergy and Immunotoxicology in Occupational Health*,
Current Topics in Environmental Health and Preventive Medicine,
DOI 10.1007/978-981-10-0351-6_9

9.1   Wide Utilization of Aluminum Nanoparticles and Concern on Their Toxicity

9.1.1   Toxicity of Aluminum

Aluminum is a very abundant metal element in the environment, comprising 8 % of the earth's crust and standing at third position in richness as elements. It is used extensively in many fields of modern life, such as industry, medicine, food, transportation, and living utensil, and may enter the human body from the environment via air, diet, drinking water, food, cosmetic, or medication. Concerns about aluminum toxicity have persisted since the demonstration as a potential neurotoxicant by Doellken more than 100 years ago [1]. This initial finding led to the extensive studies on increment of aluminum concentrations, senile plaque, and neurofibrillary tangles in the brain tissues of patients with Alzheimer's disease (AD) [2, 3]. Various mechanisms have been proposed for aluminum-induced neurotoxicity, including free-radical damage via enhanced lipid peroxidation and impaired glucose metabolism, disturbed signal transduction and protein modification, alterations in the axonal transport, and abnormal phosphorylation level of neurofilaments [4–6]. Aluminum is relatively stable in the form of alumina (aluminum oxide).

9.1.2   Chemical Property and Utilization of Nano-Al

Aluminum oxide, commonly called alumina, is a chemical compound of aluminum and oxygen with the chemical formula Al_2O_3 and is the most commonly existing type of several aluminum oxides, specifically identified as aluminum(III) oxide. It occurs in its crystalline polymorphic phase α-Al_2O_3, in which it constitutes the mineral corundum, a lot of kinds of which form the precious gemstones ruby and sapphire. Al_2O_3 is basically used to produce aluminum metal generally via electrolysis process, as an abrasive owing to its hardness and as a refractory material owing to its high melting point [7]. The nanosized form of aluminum oxide, Nano-Al, has greatly enlarged its utilization in many more industries and fields, such as transparent ceramics, cosmetics, precision polishing materials, special glass, arms, aircraft, electronics, dispersion strengthening, nanocomposites, constituent of rocket propellant, constituent of explosive for military and for mini-bomb killing cancer tissue, solar cell, and drug delivery [8]. As of October 2013, the number of consumer products of nanosized materials has increased to 1628 since 2005 [9], in which alumina is among the most abundantly produced nanosized particles; the market volume is predicted to 5000 tons only in China in 2016 [10]. With this in mind, there has been a recent emergence of concern dealing with the potential for toxicity and the lack of data to substantiate or dismiss these concerns [11–13].

9.1.3   Elevation of Concern for Toxicity of Nano-Al

Aluminum oxide was deleted from the US Environmental Protection Agency's chemicals lists in 1988, but its fibrous form is still on the EPA's Toxics Release Inventory list, and toxicity of its nanosized particles is still far from being illuminated. With so wide utilization of Nano-Al, many people, production workers, and consumers are being exposed to alumina nanoparticles occupationally and environmentally, and in living condition, concerns regarding their safety and potential toxic effect have complicated their usage. Possible adverse effect of nanosized alumina on human being's health has not been deeply investigated and elucidated, and the study on aluminum nanoparticles-induced adverse effect is rarely seen.

Toxicological studies [12, 14, 15] have shown increased toxicity of nanoparticles (<100 nm) compared to micrometer-sized particles of the same composition, which has raised concern about the impact on human health from nanoparticles.

In vitro and in vivo studies have shown that ANPs have multisystem and multiorgan toxicity on experimental animals, especially on the immune and nervous system. Thereby, we summarize the immune and neurological adverse effect of Nano-Al in this chapter based on the published data and our studies, even if the investigations were sparse.

9.1.4   Nano-Al Is Inhaled into the Respiratory System and Induces Oxidative Damage

Based on breathing air dynamics, nanosized particles can be inhaled more deeply into the respiratory system than large particles and deposited on the surface of the system. The lung tissue is considered the primary target organ for inhaled nanoparticles. Xiaobo Li et al. [16] performed H&E and TUNEL staining to detect pathology and programmed cell death in alumina nanoparticle (Al_2O_3 NPs)-exposed mice lung tissue. They found an inflammation and red blood cells located in the pulmonary mesenchyme; pneumorrhagia characterized by interstitial red blood cell distribution; massive lymphocyte infiltration, especially the subpleural area; lung cell degeneration; and massive bronchial epithelial cell apoptosis. By in vitro study using human bronchial epithelial cell (HBE cell), they also found significant increment of apoptosis ($2.24 \pm 0.17\%$), increased activities of caspase-3 and caspase-9 in Al_2O_3 NP-treated cells, indicating HBE cell apoptosis is initiated by the intrinsic apoptotic pathway, marked damage to the mitochondrial membrane potential, significantly increased cytoplasmic cytochrome c, increased reactive oxygen species (ROS) level, and increased malondialdehyde (MDA). Moreover, they also found that Al_2O_3 NPs significantly triggered downregulation of mitochondria-related genes located in complex I, IV, and V. After having damaged epithelial cells of the lung tissue, alumina NPs may be translocated from the respiratory system to other organs and systems.

Direct input into the blood compartment from the lung tissue is certainly an important translocation pathway of NPs in mammals. However, since predictive particle deposition models indicate that respiratory tract deposits alone may be far from fully accounting for the NP burden in the body, especially in the central nervous system [17], we should consider as well input from other pathways.

9.2 Immune Toxicity of Nano-Al In Vivo and In Vitro Studies

9.2.1 Aluminum NPs and Alumina NPs Damage Alveolar Macrophages and Pneumocytes with Immune Response

Alveolar macrophages are very important first frontier immune cells against foreign materials which are inhaled into the respiratory system. In an in vitro study using human alveolar macrophages (U937) and human type II pneumocytes (A549) coculture treated with aluminum nanoparticle and Al_2O_3 NPs, Laura et al. [18] found that the macrophages as frontier immune cells were more susceptible to the NPs than the epithelial cells, but if the macrophages were not present, the pneumocytes showed significant cell death, indicating that the macrophages actively engulf exotic nanoparticles and interacted with toxicity of the NPs and protected the pneumocytes. The main function of macrophages is to destroy foreign material via phagocytosis. The authors assessed if the macrophages could still phagocytose bacteria named community-acquired methicillin-resistant *Staphylococcus aureus* (ca-MRSA) after treatment with the NPs and found that the Al_2O_3 NPs did not impair phagocytosis of macrophages to the bacteria, but the Al-NPs did, meaning that the Al-NPs alter the cell function and their higher immunotoxicity than the Al_2O_3 NPs. While ca-MRSA was exposed to Al-NPs, no decrease in bacterial numbers was observed following overnight incubation, indicating that the Al-NPs do not kill this specific strain of bacteria, and the reason of Al-NP-reduced phagocytosis may be due to the Al ions released by aluminum nanoparticles, which chemically alter the cellular environment and finally disrupt the phagocytic process. In a PCR assay, Al_2O_3 NPs alone induced slightly the NF-kB pathway, but the Al-NPs did not show this induction. ca-MRSA alone generated NF-kB pathway activation in cocultured cells, but when the Al-NPs and Al_2O_3 NPs were present with ca-MRSA and together treated the coculture, the cocultured cells did not generate activation of the NF-kB pathway, indicating that the NPs are capable of altering or abolishing the cells' response to a pathogen via the NF-kB pathway. ca-MRSA infection alone induced inflammatory markers interleukin (IL)-6 and tumor necrosis factor alpha (TNF-α) response in coculture; the NPs alone did not show this effect, but while the cocultured cells were infected by ca-MRSA and the NPs were present, the expression of IL-6 and TNF-α induced by ca-MRSA was abolished, showing that the NPs inhibited ca-MRSA-induced IL-6 and TNF-α expression. In the ELISA, Al-NPs inhibited the secretion of IL-6, IL-8, IL-10, IL-1, and TNF-α too, evidencing the results of the PCR assay.

9.2.2 Alumina NP-Induced Immunotoxicity Is Complicated

In a repeated dose exposure experiment reported by Eun Jung Park et al. [19], 6-week-old male ICR mice were acclimatized for 1 week, and then Al_2O_3-NPs were administered orally at a dose of 1.5, 3, and 6 mg/kg for 13 weeks, and the control group was treated with autoclaved water. Blood (approximately 1.2 mL/mouse) was collected from the saphenous vein for biochemical and hemogram analysis, and then the mice were sacrificed, and the brain, thymus, lung, heart, liver, kidneys, spleen, and testis were collected for histological examinations. The levels of aspartate aminotransaminase (AST), alanine aminotransferase (ALT), and lactate dehydrogenase (LDH) in blood were significantly different between the Al_2O_3-NP-treated group and the controls. Compared with the controls, the levels of AST, ALT, and LDH decreased in the mice treated with 1.5 and 3 mg/kg Al_2O_3-NPs, but interestingly, these levels were markedly elevated in the 6 mg/kg Al_2O_3-NP-treated mice. In addition, with the same tendency, the accounted number of white blood cells (WBCs) and the proportion of lymphocytes in the WBCs in the mice treated with 1.5 and 3 mg/kg Al_2O_3-NPs were decreased compared with the control group, while those in the 6 mg/kg Al_2O_3-NP-treated group were significantly increased; the proportion of eosinophils in the WBCs in the mice treated with 1.5 and 3 mg/kg Al_2O_3-NPs was increased than in the control group, whereas that markedly decreased in the 6 mg/kg Al_2O_3-NP-treated group. The levels of IL-1β and TNF-α in the Al_2O_3-NP-treated groups did not show significant change compared with the control group, and granulocyte-macrophage colony-stimulating factor and transforming growth factor β were not detected at a significant level in all samples tested. However, the levels of IL-6 and monocyte chemotactic protein-1 increased in a dose-dependent manner. The results of Eun Jung Park et al. indicated that the immunotoxic effect of Nano-Al is complicated.

9.2.3 Al₂O₃ Nanoparticle Has Higher Immunotoxicity Than Micro-sized Alumina

In a 30-day Al_2O_3-NPs exposure study performed by Li Huan and colleagues [20], 70 healthy SPF ICR mice (3 months old) were treated with Al_2O_3 nanoparticle (13 nm diameter) at 25 mg/kg bw, 50 mg/kg bw, and 75 mg/kg bw as an exposure dose grade and Al_2O_3 nanoparticle (50 nm diameter) at 50 mg/kg bw and bulk Al_2O_3 at 50 mg/kg bw as comparison between nanosized alumina particle and micro-sized alumina particle, by nasal instillation, three times daily, continuously for 30 days.

Superoxide dismutase (SOD) activity and glutathione (GSH) content in the spleen tissue and thymus tissue of Al_2O_3 particle-treated mice decreased significantly compared with blank and solvent controls, and in a dose-dependent and particle size-dependent manner, i.e., the higher the dose was, and the smaller the particle size was, the higher the SOD activity and GSH contents were. While MDA content in the spleen tissue and thymus tissue of Al_2O_3 particle-treated mice increased significantly compared with blank and solvent controls, and in a dose-dependent and particle size-dependent manner, the oxidative stress level was increased with increment of doses administered with alumina nanoparticles and with decrement of particle sizes. Inflammatory cytokines IL-1α, IL-1β, interferon-γ (IFN-γ), TNF-α, IL-2, and IL-10 contents in the spleen tissue and thymus tissue increased significantly, indicating immune response in Nano-Al-treated mice was upregulated. The results of this study showed that respiratory exposure to Al_2O_3 nanoparticle could initiate oxidative stress and immune response more strongly than the controls and bigger Al_2O_3 particles, implying Al_2O_3 nanoparticle has higher immunotoxicity than micro-sized alumina.

9.3   Neurotoxicity of Nano-Al

9.3.1   Nanoalumina Induces Neurobehavioral Impairment

In an in vivo study with male ICR mice [21], Zhang et al. compared the neurotoxicity of Nano-Al and nano-carbon (Nano-C) as reference of the same particle size and different chemical property and micro-alumina (Micro-Al) as reference of the same chemical property and different particle size. The animals were inoculated intranasally (i.n.) per day with Nano-Al, Nano-C, and Micro-Al at the dose of 100 mg/kg bw as experimental groups, whereas another group of animals that received 0.9% saline were used as controls. The mice were sacrificed 10 days post-inoculation.

Tested with Morris water maze, treatment with Nano-Al dramatically lengthened the escape latency of animals (Nano-Al vs. control and Nano-C $p < 0.01$, respectively; Nano-Al vs. Micro-Al, $p < 0.05$). During the probe trial when the platform was removed, the Nano-Al-treated mice spent significantly less time in the target quadrant (Nano-Al vs. control, $p < 0.01$; Micro-Al vs. Control, $p < 0.05$) and exhibited fewer platform crossings (Nano-Al vs. control, $p < 0.01$; Micro-Al vs. Control, $p < 0.05$). In Nano-C-treated groups, both measurements were decreased but showed no significant difference from those of the control group (Nano-C vs. control, $p > 0.05$ for both parameters). In contrast, comparisons between Nano-Al- and Micro-Al-treated groups indicated that mice treated with Nano-Al required longer escape latency, spent less time in the target quadrant, and crossed the platform fewer times (Nano-Al vs. Micro-Al, $p < 0.05$). In an in vivo study with mice exposed to Nano-Al particles by the respiratory tract [22], Xin Zhang and colleagues reported that only in female mice the neurobehavioral changes and especially depression-like behavior appeared.

Yinxia Li et al. [23] observed effects of acute exposure to Al_2O_3 NPs and bulk Al_2O_3 (micro-sized) on locomotion behaviors of nematodes. After exposure for 6 h, the significant decreases in head thrashes ($p < 0.01$) and body bends ($p < 0.01$) were observed in both nematodes exposed to 51–203.9 mg/L of Al_2O_3-NPs and nematodes exposed to the same doses of bulk Al_2O_3. Nevertheless, both head thrashes and body bends in Al_2O_3-NP-exposed nematodes were lower than those in bulk Al_2O_3-exposed nematodes. Moreover, after exposure for 48 h, the similar but more deteriorated locomotion behaviors were observed. The authors further examined the 10-day chronic neurotoxicity from 8.1 to 23.1 mg/L of Al_2O_3-NPs and same doses of bulk Al_2O_3 exposure on locomotion behavior of nematodes and got the similar results as the acute exposure experiment got. The authors concluded that Al_2O_3-NPs are more neurotoxic than bulk Al_2O_3, implying that alumina nanoparticles possess higher neurotoxicity than micro-sized alumina particles.

9.3.2 Inhaled Particles May Enter into the Central Nervous System via Mainly Two Routs: Blood Circulation and Olfactory Nerve

Chen Lei et al. [24] injected Alizarin Red S-labeled nanoalumina at the dose of 1.25 mg/kg into the mouse cerebral circulation via the carotid artery and detected the brain endothelium and astrocytes by staining for factor VIII as endothelium marker and GFAP as astrocyte marker, respectively. They found that Alizarin Red S-labeled-nanoalumina particles were colocalized with the brain endothelium 1 h after injection and were also appeared in astrocytes surrounding the cerebral vessels. Twenty-four hours after injection, Alizarin Red S-labeled-nanoalumina particles were diffused in brain parenchyma close to astrocytes. The distribution pattern of Alizarin Red S-labeled-nanoalumina particles in one week after injection was similar to that in 24 h after injection, indicating that nanoalumina particles passed the blood-brain barrier, entered into the brain tissue, and accumulated in the brain and not eliminated from the brain components. In order to examine how the nanoalumina particles impaired the BBB, the author further assessed the effects of nanoalumina on the levels of occludin and claudin-5, two types of important tight-junction proteins that regulate integrity and barrier function of the brain endothelium, in human cerebral microvascular endothelial cells (HCMECs). Following a 6-h exposure to nanoalumina, a dose-dependent decrease in expression of occludin and claudin-5 expression was detected in HCMECs. Nanoalumina also decreased tight-junction protein expression in vivo. A single dose of nanoalumina (1.25 mg/kg) was administered to mouse via the carotid artery, a gradual decrease in occludin for up to 30 days after injection was observed. Injection with 1.25 mg/kg nanoalumina significantly elevated blood-brain barrier permeability at day 3 after injection, and this effect was preserved for up to 30 days, indicating that only a single intravascular nanoalumina exposure can damage the BBB and the effect can last up to 30 days, and even the exposure dose is not high.

Though there was not a report on other pathways of Nano-Al entering the brain tissue except for blood circulation, there was a report on Nano-C entering the brain tissue via the olfactory nerve. Oberdörster et al. [25] exposed rats with Nano-C particles (36 nm) for 6 h, sacrificed the rats, and removed and examined the lungs, cerebrum, cerebellum, and olfactory bulbs of exposed rats at 1, 3, 5, and 7 days after exposure. The concentration of Nano-C particles in the lung tissue decreased from 1.39 µg/g on day 1 to 0.59 µg/g by day 7 after exposure, but the Nano-C particles in the olfactory bulb significantly and persistently increased, from 0.35 µg/g on day 1 to 0.43 µg/g by day 7, implying that the olfactory nerve is a channel for Nano-C entering into the brain tissue. Based on this fact, the authors concluded that the CNS can be targeted by airborne nanoparticles and that the most likely mechanism is from deposits on the olfactory mucosa of the nasopharyngeal region of the respiratory tract to subsequent translocation via the olfactory nerve. Depending on particle size, more than 50 % of inhaled nanoparticles can be deposited in the nasopharyngeal region during nasal breathing. The authors estimated that approximately 20 % of the nanoparticles deposited on the olfactory mucosa of the rat can be translocated to the olfactory bulb and then into other parts of the brain tissue. The increases of carbon nanoparticles in olfactory bulbs are consistent with studies in rodents that demonstrated that intranasally instilled solid ultrafine elemental particle translocates along axons of the olfactory nerve into the CNS [26].

9.3.3 Nanoalumina Induces Cerebrovascular Damage via Autophagy

In an in vitro *study* performed by Lei Chen [24], HCMECs were treated with Alizarin Red S-labeled nanoalumina (1 µg/mL) for 6 h and stained with MitoTracker Red, MitoTracker Green, and MDC (marker for autophagic vacuoles). Alizarin Red S-labeled nanoalumina (1 µg/mL, stained red) was detected in HCMECs following a 2-h treatment. After a 12-h exposure, Alizarin Red S-labeled nanoalumina was visible as aggregates close to clustered mitochondria stained by MitoTracker Green, which indicates the loss of mitochondria membrane potential, and a notable increase of MDC intensity indicates enhanced autophagy.

In a same in vivo *study* performed by Chen Lei [24] described in Sect. 4.2, nanoalumina (1.25 mg/kg) was administered to mouse via the carotid artery, and 24 h later, mouse brains were taken out and subjected to mouse autophagy PCR array, and 84 autophagy-related genes were examined; 13 autophagy-related genes increased more than twofold. Then two frequently used autophagy marker proteins LC3 and p62 were also examined. Similar to the results obtained in HCMECs, in which a notable increase of MDC intensity showed an increased autophagy, an increase in LC3 and p62 proteins, which indicate autophagy too, was observed 24 h after nanoalumina injection and remained elevated for as long as 30 days after nanoalumina administration. Combining Chen Lei's results, we could hypothesize that

Nano-Al particles preserve continuously in blood circulation compartment and damage the BBB and are difficult to be discharged from circulation compartment and the brain tissue.

The effects of nanoalumina on protein degradation were assessed in HCMECs using DQ-BSA, a probe based on bovine serum albumin (BSA) labeled with red fluorescent BODIPY TR-X dye (Invitrogen). Treatment with nanoalumina dose-dependently elevated activity of DQ-fluorescence, and protein degradation activity was correlated with the formation of acidic vesicles, consistent with autophagolysosomes stained with LysoTracker Green.

9.3.4 Nano-Al Induces Neural Cell Death

In the same in vivo study as in Sect. 4.1 with male ICR mice [21], Zhang et al. compared the neurotoxicity of Nano-Al and Nano-C as reference of the same particle size and different chemical property and Micro-Al as reference of the same chemical property and different particle size. The animals were inoculated intranasally (i.n.) per day with Nano-Al, Nano-C, and Micro-Al at the dose of 100 mg/kg bw as experimental groups, whereas another group of animals that received 0.9 % saline were used as controls. The mice were sacrificed 10 days post-inoculation.

To investigate the potential mechanisms by which Nano-Al more strongly impaired the neurobehavior of animals than Nano-C and Micro-Al did, the changes in matrix metalloprotein (MMP) and ROS were observed. Treatment with 100 mg/kg Nano-Al but not with the same concentration of Nano-C resulted in a highly significant decrease in MMP. Alterations in mitochondrial potential may result in induction of cellular oxidative stress; indeed, ROS production measurements showed that Nano-Al led to a marked induction of oxidative stress.

Nano-Al-mediated MMP loss and significantly higher ROS production confirmed that Nano-Al may cause more severe neurotoxicity than Micro-Al. On the other hand, Nano-C with the same nanoparticle size resulted in only mild neurotoxicity that was not significantly different compared with controls treated with 0.9 % saline.

Both Nano-C and Nano-Al at 100 mg/kg bw were toxic and enhanced the necrotic rate, and the necrotic rate induced by Nano-Al was markedly higher than apoptotic rate it induced. Apoptosis was also observed in Nano-Al-treated mice and became more pronounced in Micro-Al-treated mice.

LC3 is a mammalian homolog of yeast Atg8, the only reliable marker of autophagosomes that indicate autophagy process. In order to recognize if autophagy exists in nanoparticle-induced neurotoxicity, the authors observed LC3 expression in the study and found its expression was low.

Lower expression of LC3 in the study suggests that autophagy may not be the major cell death mode in neural cells induced by Nano-C, Nano-Al, and Micro-Al. Furthermore, robust caspase-3 activation likely indicates significant apoptosis in Micro-Al-treated mice. The results also indicated that Nano-Al treatment led to neural cell death; and necrosis may be a major cell death mode in nanoparticle-induced neurotoxicity.

Furthermore, in an in vitro study performed by Zhang et al. [27], observed under light microscope, neural cells treated with Micro-Al presented shrink and irregular shape, indicating apoptotic-like cell death, while Nano-C particle-treated cells exhibited blackish color, flat, and swelling shape in cell body, indicating necrotic-like cell death. The Nano-C particles with the same size as Nano-Al could enter into the cell body and accumulate in the cell cytoplasma. Whereas treated by Nano-Al particles with the same chemical composition of Micro-Al and the same size with Nano-C, the neural cells displayed morphological characteristics of both Nano-C- and Micro-Al-treated cells, presenting both brownish particle accumulation and condensed nuclei and cell organelle disrupture and necrotic cell death.

Under transmission electron microscope, margination of condensed chromatin appeared in the Micro-Al-treated cells; the Nano-C-treated cells displayed nanoparticles inside the cytoplasma and nucleus, indicating the disrupture of cellular and nucleus membrane, while Nano-C-treated cells manifested the nanoparticles inside the cytoplasma with disrupted cell membrane, chromatin aggregation, and broken fragments surrounded by dissolved cytoplasma and organelles, indicating presentation of both the Nano-C- and Micro-Al-induced cell impairment features. Endocytosis appeared in Nano-Al-treated cells, and the cell bodies and their nuclei seemed to be disrupted and dissolved in the presence of the Nano-Al particles. Nanoparticles of alumina are located in the primary lysosome, secondary lysosome, and accumulated lysosomes in neural cells. The cell viability in Nano-Al-exposed cells was much lower than those in Micro-Al- and Nano-C-exposed cells ($p < 0.05$, $p < 0.01$). However, there was no significant difference between the viabilities of cells treated with Nano-C and Micro-Al ($p > 0.05$).

9.3.5 Aluminum Nanoparticles Induce Activation of MAPK Signal Pathway or Inhibit It

In a study performed by Jung-Taek Kwon [28], rats were exposed to Al-NPs by nasal instillation at 1 mg/kg body weight (low exposure group), 20 mg/kg body weight (moderate exposure group), and 40 mg/kg body weight (high exposure group), for a total of three times, with a 24-h interval after each exposure. Inductively coupled plasma mass spectrometry (ICP-MS) analysis indicated that the presence of aluminum in the olfactory bulb and the brain of Al-NP-treated mice was increased dose dependently. In microarray analysis, the regulation of mitogen-activated protein kinase (MAPK) activity was significantly overexpressed in the Al-NP-treated mice than in the controls ($p = 0.0027$). Moreover, Al-NPs induced the activation of ERK1 and p38 MAPK protein expression in the brain, but did not alter the protein expression of JNK, when compared with the controls. The results demonstrate that the nasal exposure of Al-NPs can permeate the brain via the olfactory bulb and modulate the gene and protein expression of MAPK and its activity. But another study confirmed that Al-NP exposure activated the JNK pathway [29].

But, in another study [30], the effect of Nano-Al on brain energy metabolism was evaluated in alumina NP-treated and NP-untreated mouse brain homogenates via western blot. The results indicated that Nano-Al inactivated MAPK and dephosphorylated it at Thr172 and reduced the expression of AMP-activated protein kinase (AMPK) in the brain compared to the untreated mice, while the total AMPK level remained unchanged. Similarly, the AMPK activity was also reduced in the brain homogenates of Nano-Al-treated mice analyzed through the CycLex® AMPK activity assay method. Additionally, the expression of p-AMPK was measured via immunofluorescence in the hippocampal cornu ammonis 1 (CA1) and cortical regions of nanoalumina-treated and nanoalumina-untreated mice. The images of immunofluorescence revealed that nanoalumina significantly inhibited the expression of p-AMPK, which supported western blot results, suggesting that alumina nanoparticles are involved in the disturbance of brain energy metabolism.

9.3.6 Nano-Al Can Induce Oxidative Stress in Neural Cells Both In Vitro and In Vivo

To analyze whether mouse hippocampal neural cell line, HT22 cells, can take up Nano-Al and increase their aluminum level, morin staining was performed in the same study as Sect. 4.5 [30]. Exposure of HT22 cells to Nano-Al caused an increased uptake of Nano-Al, which ultimately increased the aluminum abundance in cultured HT22 cells. Furthermore, to assess whether Nano-Al induces oxidative stress in HT22 cells, 8-oxo-guanine (8-OxoG) staining was performed using an anti-8-OxoG monoclonal antibody. The immunofluorescence images show that Nano-Al induced oxidative stress and produced a significantly high number of ROS in the Al-NP-treated HT22 cells in contrast to untreated HT22 cells.

In an in vivo *study* performed by the same authors, Nano-Al was peripherally administered to ICR female mice for three weeks. The immunohistological evaluations for abundance of brain aluminum were conducted in the hippocampal CA1, CA3, and dentate gyrus (DG) and cortical regions of the female mouse brain. The results indicated that exogenously administered nanoalumina significantly increased brain aluminum abundance compared with the untreated control mice. In vivo 8-OxoG staining was performed to analyze the extent of oxidative stress induced by nanoalumina, and it was evident from the immunostaining images that Nano-Al induced oxidative stress by increasing 8-OxoG expression in the brains of Al-NP-exposed mice. This trend was mainly observed in different parts of the hippocampus including CA1 and CA3, respectively, and DG and the cortical regions in Al-NP-treated mice, while no or only a few 8-OxoG appearances were seen in the hippocampus and cortical regions in the untreated control mice.

9.3.7 Nano-Al Can Induce Aβ Production via Amyloidogenic Pathway in Mice

The same authors of Sect. 4.6 study further to investigate Aβ production via the amyloidogenic pathway as a consequence of Nano-Al treatment in mice. The western blot results showed that the administration of nanoparticles to mice enhanced the amyloidogenic pathway of Aβ production. Nano-Al upregulated the expression of the amyloid precursor protein (APP) and β-secretase beta-site amyloid precursor protein cleaving enzyme 1 (BACE1) activity, which significantly increased the generation of Aβ in treated mice compared with untreated controls. Moreover, it also caused downregulation of the α-secretase enzyme sAPP-α, which is responsible for the generation of nontoxic Aβ peptides through a non-amyloidogenic pathway. The levels of soluble Aβ1–42 in the brain homogenates were measured through the ELISA method and revealed that Nano-Al significantly increased the production of Aβ1–42. Interestingly, Nano-Al also caused the formation of Aβ aggregation and plaques in the hippocampus and cortical regions of the brain in Al-NP-treated mice, which was measured immunohistopathologically both via the Aβ (6E10) antibody and thioflavin S staining. The effect of increase in the Aβ level produced by Nano-Al on the hyperphosphorylation of microtubule-associated tau at ser413 and synapse related proteins, including synaptophysin and postsynapse density protein 95 (PSD 95), was investigated via western blot. The result indicated that Aβ induced a significant increase in the expression level of p-tau (while the total tau protein level was unchanged) and downregulated the expression of synaptophysin and PSD 95 proteins in treated mice compared to the controls.

9.3.8 Nano-Al Induced Neurodegeneration In Vivo

The toxic effect of the administered Nano-Al on inducing neurodegeneration was further examined by Shahid Ali Shah, who analyzed the expression of apoptotic markers via western blot. The results indicated that Nano-Al significantly upregulated the expression of various apoptotic markers or apoptotic signals, such as cleaved caspase-3 and cleaved PARP-1, in the hippocampus and cortical sections of the mouse brain. However, caspase-3 and PARP-1 were less expressed in untreated mice. Additionally, Fluoro-Jade B (FJB) staining was performed to investigate the neurodegeneration in the hippocampus and cortical regions in mice by the administered Nano-Al. The staining of the cortical and hippocampal CA1, CA3, and DG regions of nanoalumina-treated mice revealed that the alumina nanoparticles induced neuronal cell death, as was evidenced by the number of positive FJB cells, whereas no such positive stainings were observed in the brain sections of the control mouse.

References

1. Doelken V. Ueber die wirkung des aluminiums mit besonderer berucksichtigung der durch das aluminium verursachten lasionen im centralnerven-system. Arch Exp Pathol Pharmakol. 1898;40:98–120.
2. Frisardi V, Solfrizzi V, Capurso C, Kehoe PG, Imbimbo BP, Santamato A, Dellegrazie F, Seripa D, Pilotto A, Capurso A, Panza F. Aluminum in the diet and Alzheimer's disease: from current epidemiology to possible disease-modifying treatment. J Alzheimers Dis. 2010;20(1):17–30.
3. Walton JR. Brain lesions comprised of aluminum-rich cells that lack microtubules may be associated with the cognitive deficit of Alzheimer's disease. Neurotoxicology. 2009;30(6):1059–69.
4. Esparza JL, Gomez M, Romeu MR, Mulero M, Sanchez DJ, Mallol J, Domingo JL. Melatonin reduces oxidative stress and increases gene expression in the cerebral cortex and cerebellum of aluminum-exposed rats. J Pineal Res. 2005;39(2):129–36.
5. Walton JR. An aluminum-based rat model for Alzheimer's disease exhibits oxidative damage, inhibition of PP2A activity, hyperphosphorylated tau, and granulovacuolar degeneration. J Inorg Biochem. 2007;101(9):1275–84.
6. Gupta VB, Anitha S, Hegde ML, Zecca L, Garruto RM, Ravid R, Shankar SK, Stein R, Shanmugavelu P, Jagannatha Rao KS. Aluminium in Alzheimer's disease: are we still at a crossroad? Cell Mol Life Sci. 2005;62(2):143–58.
7. Dörre E, Hübner H. Alumina processing, properties, and applications. Berlin: Springer; 1984.
8. Meziani MJ, Bunker CE, Lu F, Li H, Wang W, Guliants EA, Quinn RA, Sun YP. Formation and properties of stabilized aluminum nanoparticles. ACS Appl Mater Interfaces. 2009;1(3):703–9.
9. Nanotechnology – Project on Emerging Nanotechnologies. Inventory FindsIncrease in Consumer Products Containing Nanoscale Materials [http://www.nanotechproject.org/inventories/consumer/updates/]. Date accessed: 28 Apr 2016.
10. Feasibility analysis and development tendency prediction of nano-alumina projects in China and World (2016 edition) http://www.baogaochina.com/List_YeJinBaoGao/33/NaMiYangHuaLvHangYeXianZhuangYuFaZhanQianJing.html
11. Maynard AD. Nanotechnology: the next big thing, or much ado about nothing? Ann Occup Hyg. 2007;51(1):1–12.
12. Stanley JK, Coleman JG, Weiss CA, Steevens JA. Sediment toxicity and bioaccumulation of nano and micron-sized aluminum oxide. Environ Toxicol Chem. 2010;29(2):422–9.
13. Balasubramanyam A, Sailaja N, Mahboob M, Rahman MF, Hussain SM, Grover P. In vitro mutagenicity assessment of aluminium oxide nanomaterials using the Salmonella/microsome assay. Toxicol In Vitro. 2010;24(6):1871–6.
14. McLeish JA, Chico TJ, Taylor HB, Tucker C, Donaldson K, Brown SB. Skin exposure to micro- and nano-particles can cause haemostasis in zebrafish larvae. Thromb Haemost. 2011;103(4):797–807.
15. Jiang W, Mashayekhi H, Xing B. Bacterial toxicity comparison between nano- and micro-scaled oxide particles. Environ Pollut. 2009;157(5):1619–25.
16. Li X, Zhang C, Zhang X, Wang S, Meng Q, Wu S, Yang H, Xia Y, Chen R. An acetyl-L-carnitine switch on mitochondrial dysfunction and rescue in the metabolomics study on aluminum oxide nanoparticles. Part Fibre Toxicol. 2016;13:4. doi:10.1186/s12989-016-0115-y.
17. Oberdörster G, Sharp Z, Atudorei V, Elder A, Gelein R, Lunts A, Kreyling W, Cox C. Extrapulmonary translocation of ultrafine carbon particles following whole-body inhalation exposure of rats. J Toxicol Environ Health A. 2002;65(20):1531–43.
18. Braydich-Stolle LK, Speshock JL, Castle A, Smith M, Murdock RC, Hussain SM. Nanosized aluminum altered immune function. ACS Nano. 2010;4(7):3661–70.

19. Park EJ, Sim J, Kim Y, Han BS, Yoon C, Lee S, Cho MH, Lee BS, Kim JH. A 13 week repeated dose oral toxicity and bioaccumulation of aluminum oxide nanoparticles in mice. Arch Toxicol. 2015;89:371–9.
20. Huan L, Yong D, Xiaohong W, Yaxian P, Cuicui G, Wang H, Wenhui W, Qi Z, Qiao N, Qinli Z. Impact of Nano-alumina particles on variations of immune indices in mice. J Toxicol. 2015;29(2):114–8.
21. Zhang QL, Li MQ, Ji JW, Gao FP, Bai R, Chen CY, Wang ZW, Zhang C, Niu Q. *in vivo* toxicity of nano-alumina on mice neurobehavioral profiles and the potential mechanisms. Int J Immunopathol Pharmacol. 2011;24(1S):23–9.
22. Zhang X, Xu Y, Zhou L, Zhang C, Meng Q, Wu S, Wang S, Ding Z, Chen X, Li X, Chen R. Sex-dependent depression-like behavior induced by respiratory administration of aluminum oxide nanoparticles. Int J Environ Res Public Health. 2015;12(12):15692–705.
23. Yinxia L, Shunhui Y, Quili W, Meng T, Yuepu P, Dayong W. Chronic Al_2O_3-nanoparticle exposure causes neurotoxic effects on locomotion behaviors by inducing severe ROS production and disruption of ROS defense mechanisms in nematode Caenorhabditis elegans. J Hazard Mater. 2012;219– 220:221–30.
24. Chen L, Yokel RA, Hennig B, Toborek M. Manufactured aluminum oxide nanoparticles decrease expression of tight junction proteins in brain vasculature. J Neuroimmune Pharmacol. 2008;3:286–95.
25. Oberdörster G, Sharp Z, Atudorei V, Elder A, Gelein R, Kreyling W, Cox C. Translocation of inhaled ultrafine particles to the brain. Inhal Toxicol. 2004;16(6–7):437–45.
26. Wang B, Feng WY, Wang M, Shi JW, Zhang F, Ouyang H, Zhao YL, Chai ZF, Huang YY, Xie YN, Wang HF, Wang J. Transport of intranasally instilled fine Fe_2O_3 particles into the brain: micro-distribution, chemical states, and histopathological observation. Biol Trace Elem Res. 2007;118(3):233–43.
27. Zhang Q, Xu L, Wang J, Sabbioni E, Piao L, Di Gioacchino M, Niu Q. Lysosomes involved in the cellular toxicity of nano-alumina: combined effects of particle size and chemical composition. J Biol Regul Homeost Agents. 2013;27(2):365–75.
28. Kwon J-T, Seo G-B, Jo E, Lee M, Kim H-M, Shim I, Lee B-W, Yoon B-I, Kim P, Choi K. Aluminum nanoparticles induce ERK and p38MAPK activation in rat brain. Toxicol Res. 2013;29(3):181–5.
29. Kleinmana MT, Araujob J, Nelc A, Sioutasd C, Campbelle A, Conga PQ, Lia H, Bondya SC. Inhaled ultrafine particulate matter affects CNS inflammatory processes and may act via MAP kinase signaling pathways. Toxicol Lett. 2008;178(2):127–30.
30. Shah SA, Yoon GH, Ahmad A, Ullah F, Ul Amin F, Kim MO. Nanoscale-alumina induces oxidative stress and accelerates amyloid beta (Aβ) production in ICR female mice. Nanoscale. 2015;7:15225.

Chapter 10
Non Pulmonary Effects of Isocyanates

Paola Pedata, Anna Rita Corvino, Monica Lamberti, Claudia Petrarca, Luca Di Giampaolo, Nicola Sannolo, and Mario Di Gioacchino

Abstract Isocyanates are highly reactive compounds of low molecular weight containing the functional group –N=C=O. Isocyanates are increasingly used in the fabrication of many products such as elastomers, paints, adhesive, coating, insecticides, and resins with a variety of industrial applications after polymerization with alcohols to form polyurethanes. The high chemical reactivity of isocyanates, an important characteristic in industrial applications, also makes them toxic products. Isocyanates currently are the most commonly identified cause of occupational asthma in industrialized countries. Exposure to diisocyanates, polyisocyanates, and polyurethane additives may also cause allergic and irritant contact dermatitis (ACD, ICD) and may result in neurotoxic and carcinogenic effects.

The purpose of this paper is to review and synthesize the literature regarding non-pulmonary health effects of isocyanates to address several key unresolved

P. Pedata (✉) • A.R. Corvino • M. Lamberti • N. Sannolo
Department of Experimental Medicine, Section of Hygiene, Occupational Medicine and Forensic Medicine, Second University of Naples, Naples, Italy
e-mail: paola.pedata@unina2.it

C. Petrarca
Immuntotoxicology and Allergy Unit & Occupational Biorepository,
Center of Excellence on Aging and Translational Medicine (CeSI-MeT), "G. D'Annunzio" University Foundation, Chieti, Italy

L. Di Giampaolo
Department of Medical Oral and Biotechnological Science, G. d'Annunzio University, Chieti, Italy

M. Di Gioacchino
Immuntotoxicology and Allergy Unit & Occupational Biorepository,
Center of Excellence on Aging and Translational Medicine (CeSI-MeT), "G. D'Annunzio" University Foundation, Chieti, Italy

Department of Medicine and Science of Aging, G. d'Annunzio University, Chieti, Italy

© Springer Science+Business Media Singapore 2017
T. Otsuki et al. (eds.), *Allergy and Immunotoxicology in Occupational Health*,
Current Topics in Environmental Health and Preventive Medicine,
DOI 10.1007/978-981-10-0351-6_10

129

issues, including the carcinogenic and neurotoxic effects, and to focus on the often unrecognized skin effects.

Keywords Isocyanates • Health effects • Carcinogenic effects • Neurotoxic effects • Skin effects

10.1 Introduction

Isocyanates are highly reactive compounds of low molecular weight containing the functional group $-N=C=O$.

Isocyanates are classified, based on number of $N=C=O$ groups in the molecules, into monoisocyanates (one NCO), diisocyanates (two NCO), or polyisocyanates (multiple NCOs). In diisocyanate, the two functional groups can directly polymerize with alcohols to form polyurethanes, resins with a variety of industrial applications. Polyisocyanates represent the major source of exposure to isocyanate groups in many workplaces, and like the diisocyanate monomers from which they are derived, such as toluene diisocyanate (TDI), diphenylmethane diisocyanate (MDI), and hexamethylene diisocyanate (HDI), they are increasingly used in the production of elastomers, paints, adhesives, coatings, insecticides, and many other products.

Aliphatic isocyanates such as those based on HDI are used mostly in external paints and coatings because of their excellent resistance to chemicals and abrasion and superior weathering characteristics such as gloss and color retention.

Aromatic isocyanates, such as MDI, are used in many applications such as foams, adhesives, sealants, elastomers and binders, which require fast curing rates and have less stringent requirements on their chemical and mechanical stability.

Polyurethane foams are a major end use of aromatic isocyanates [1]. There are several reports of sensitization to polyurethane products also in a domestic setting, such as to a plastic watchstrap, spectacle frames, and a pacemaker lining due to the increasing popularity of "do it yourself"; for this reason, isocyanates are likely to become more common chemicals within houses [2].

The high chemical reactivity of isocyanates, an important characteristic in their industrial use, also makes them toxic. Despite substantial research on isocyanates, the pathogenic mechanisms, host susceptibility factors, and dose-response relationships remain unclear [3–5]. Isocyanates can bind to carrier proteins, via the reaction of the NCO group with nucleophiles such as SH, NH_2, NH, and OH groups present on these proteins. Several peptides and proteins found in airway epithelial cells, serum, and skin have been observed to bind diisocyanates, including glutathione [6, 7], albumin [8, 9], tubulin [10], and keratin [9, 11]. Covalent binding of isocyanate groups to carrier proteins is likely an important step in the chain of events leading to health effects, in particular sensitization and asthma [1].

Respiratory exposure to isocyanates has long been considered the primary way of exposure, and thus, research, regulation, and prevention have focused almost exclusively on airborne isocyanate exposures [12]. However, respiratory exposures have been reduced through improved hygiene controls and the use of less-volatile isocyanates [1], thus potentially increasing the relative importance of skin exposure. Numerous isocyanate end uses, such as spraying and application of foams and adhesives, may cause isocyanate skin exposure from deposition of aerosols and/or absorption of vapors. Typical workplace isocyanate exposure levels are not irritating and give few warning signs and skin protective equipment may not be worn, even when respiratory protection is used [13]. Skin exposure is the consequence of direct contact of unprotected skin or the failure of personal protective equipments, like gloves; particularly events such as spills, cleanup, and contact with contaminated equipments represent the major opportunities for isocyanate skin exposure. There are some investigations showing that isocyanates [14] and solvents [15] can be detected underneath gloves.

Isocyanate skin exposure could contribute a significant part of the total body burden. Multiple lines of evidence from animal studies and clinical, epidemiologic, and biomarker studies, as well as anecdotal evidence, suggest that in certain exposure setting, human skin likely is an important route of isocyanate exposure and can contribute to the development of isocyanate health effects [16].

Isocyanates currently are the most commonly identified cause of occupational asthma in industrialized countries, where its prevalence among exposed workers ranges from 1 % to even 25 %. These chemicals were also reported as causal factors of other respiratory disorders as nonobstructive bronchitis, rhinitis, chronic obstructive pulmonary disease, and less commonly extrinsic allergic alveolitis [16, 17].

Several observations suggest that skin exposure occurs and can contribute to the development of isocyanate asthma presumably by inducing systemic sensitization. In fact, isocyanate respiratory exposure alone, without any skin exposure, seems unlikely in most work settings. Isocyanate asthma occurs in settings with minimal documented respiratory exposures but clear potential for skin exposure, and splashes and spills have been reported by workers who subsequently develop isocyanate asthma [18–22].

Exposure to diisocyanates, polyisocyanates, and polyurethane additives may also cause allergic and irritant contact dermatitis [23]. Contact hypersensitivity (allergic contact dermatitis) following skin exposure to isocyanates is well documented in animals and in clinical dermatologic literature, with sensitization confirmed with patch testing [24, 25]. Allergic contact dermatitis has been reported following skin exposure to isocyanates and polyurethane products in a number of different workplace and non-occupational settings, but has not been considered common and is rarely reported in workers with isocyanate asthma [24, 26–28]. However, allergic contact dermatitis may be more common than suspected because symptoms can be mild, workers being evaluated for asthma are frequently not asked about skin problems, and patch testing can be falsely negative [24, 29].

Another potential health disease related to exposure to isocyanates are neurotoxic effects consisting in lightheadedness, headache, insomnia, mental aberrations, impaired gait, loss of consciousness, and coma due to acute exposure and alterations in the central and peripheral nervous systems for chronic exposure. Moreover, a systematic review of the literature evaluating the causal association on humans does not exist to support this alleged association [30].

Another open question is whether occupational isocyanate exposure is a carcinogenic hazard. TDI has been classified as carcinogenic in animals on the basis of gavage administration studies, but no conclusions are available on inhalation exposure. TDI is classified as a Group 2B carcinogen (possibly carcinogenic to humans) by the International Agency for Research on Cancer (IARC) [31] and as an A4 carcinogen (not classifiable as a human carcinogen) by the American Conference of Governmental Industrial Hygienists (ACGIH) [32]. For MDI, there is suggestive evidence for carcinogenicity in rats. Both chemicals have been positive in a number of short-term tests inducing gene mutations and chromosomal damage [33].

Over the past several years, there has been an increasing collection of clinical and epidemiologic data related to isocyanate health effects, especially those regarding respiratory ones, although knowledge and awareness remain limited regarding the non-pulmonary effects of isocyanates and some clinical studies are still unrecognized. Our purpose in this paper is to review and synthesize the literature regarding non-pulmonary effects of isocyanates to address several key unresolved issues, including the carcinogenic and neurotoxic effects of isocyanates, and to focus on the often unrecognized skin effects.

10.2   Literature Search

We selected the most relevant contributions to the literature in clinical and epidemiologic fields starting with the information retrieved from PubMed (http://www.ncbi.nlm.nih.gov/pubmed/), Google Scholar (http://scholar.google.com), and ScienceDirect (www.sciencedirect.com) using the following keywords: "isocyanates" OR "diisocyanates" OR "MDI" OR "TDI" OR "HDI", AND "health effects", AND "skin disease" OR "sensitization", AND "cancerogenesis" AND "neurotoxicity", and other synonymous terms and our own extensive collection of isocyanate publications. Additional papers were identified from the reference lists of the selected relevant articles.

The search yielded about 110 articles which were further reviewed; at the end of this selection process, 82 articles were deemed relevant to this review and were examined with a particular emphasis on non-pulmonary effects of isocyanates, such as skin diseases and neurotoxic and carcinogenic effects.

10.3   Health Effects

10.3.1   Skin Diseases

The isocyanates are an important cause of occupational asthma, but descriptions of ACD and ICD due to them are relatively uncommon [24]. In a mouse local lymph node assay examining the dermal sensitization potential of TDI, Woolhiser et al. [34] reported irritation at the TDI application site [34]. Second, Arnold et al. [35] reported that the animal studies are insufficient to characterize the dermal irritation potential of TDI due to the lack of documentation and use of nonstandard methodology; the overall weight of evidence indicates that TDI is irritating to the skin of experimental animals [35].

ACD caused by isocyanates has been reported mainly in connection with occupational exposure in the manufacture of polyurethane products used in the plastics, car and textile industries, flooring, and the manufacture of medical, electronic, and foam products. It has also been reported in sculptors [36] and a molders [37], although there is still limited knowledge about the skin diseases in occupational setting because the fact that most studies to date have been cross-sectional in design, small in size, or based on selected clinical cases or production workers rather than end use workers.

One of the first investigations on the skin effects of polyurethane products is that of Emmet et al.; this study reported skin rashes on exposed skin areas in eight workers of polyurethane molding plant, with positive patch test reactions to dicyclohexylmethane-4,4'-diisocyanate (DMDI, synonymous with hydrogenated methylene-4,4'-diphenyl diisocyanate – HDI) and diaminodiphenylmethane (MDA) in two of them [38]. White et al. showed ACD and ICD due to DMDI in uncured resin in a factory of car badges [39]. Frick et al. demonstrated ACD in workers of a company manufacturing flooring laminate boards, after the introduction of a water-repellent lacquer based on MDI. Five workers, engaged as machine operators where lacquer was sprayed onto the boards, developed eczematous lesions of the forearms, hands, or arms. Patch testing showed positive reactions to MDA in four, to MDI in one, to HDMI in one, and to a lacquer in three of them [40]. Another study of Frick et al. reported severe eczema in 17 workers exposed to glue based on DMDI, at a factory manufacturing medical equipment. Contact allergy to DMDI, other isocyanates, and/or MDA was demonstrated in 13 individuals [27].

Isolated cases of ACD in workers exposed to MDI were also reported in different occupational environment. Hannu et al. demonstrated a case of ACD due to MDI and MDA from accidental occupational exposure in a female worker of a manufacturing plant of electronic components [41]. Schroder reported a case of ACD to MDI, present in polyurethane adhesive, TDI, MDA, and epoxy resin in a female engaged in a plant manufacturing grinding tools [42]. Estlander et al. diagnosed occupational contact dermatitis in three workers exposed to MDI present, respectively, in a hardener of core binder, a hardener of adhesive, and a laboratory mixture of diisocyanates [43]. Lidén reported a case of ACD of the forearms in a molder exposed to MDI-containing product in a hospital [37]. Tait and Delaney reported a case of a maintenance fitter who developed ACD after cleaning filters contaminated with aptane isocyanate based on MDI [44]. Kerre reports a patient who developed an acute allergic contact dermatitis using a DMDI-charged cartridge to create resin-coated "3D labels" within an office environment [45].

According to Aalto-Korte et al. who analyzed 54 cases of ACD due to monomeric isocyanates, motor vehicle industry was among the most significant occupational fields for isocyanate contact allergy. They identified many sources of allergy to MDI such as polyurethane foam used in the production of car insulation material, pistol foam containing MDI, and uncured polyurethane insulation material [46]. A recent study of Kiec-Swierczynska et al. in a vehicle equipment factory revealed work-related contact dermatitis in 12 workers exposed to polyurethane foam containing MDI. Seven of them developed contact allergy to MDA and were diagnosed with occupational ACD. Irritant skin reactions to the antiadhesive agent were also observed, in three cases coexisting with occupational ACD [47].

There are several reports of sensitization to polyurethane products also in domestic setting, such as to a plastic watchstraps [26], spectacle frames [48], a pacemaker lining [49], and do-it-yourself products used for renovating objects [2], though only one of these reports has been specifically identified, sensitization to 1,6-hexamethylene diisocyanate. It is also described a case of allergic contact dermatitis caused by isocyanates, specifically DMDI, in resin jewelry making. Furthermore, this is not occupational related [50].

Isocyanates causing allergy contact dermatitis included MDI [24, 37, 41–43], TDI [24], HDI [24, 51], and DMDI [27, 39, 45, 52, 53]. Allergy contact dermatitis due to MDI was seen more frequently than that related to other isocyanates, which may be a consequence of the fact that MDI represents more than a half of the worldwide isocyanate production [46].

Occupational allergic contact dermatitis usually develops after months or years of exposure. However, strong allergens may sensitize after a single exposure [54]. According to Kanerva et al., one can assume that sensitization from a single exposure has taken place when a patient, with no previous eczema, develops the first skin symptoms soon after accidental exposure and patch testing with the chemical provokes an allergic reaction.

The most common locations of occupational dermatitis are generally the hands and forearms, but the face is also commonly affected. In a report from a general dermatology clinic, facial symptoms were more common among TDI-positive or isophorone diisocyanate (IPDI)-positive cases than among MDA-positive or MDI-positive ones [55]. Although in later investigations no difference was noted when MDI-positive patients were compared with IPDI-positive or TDI-positive cases, facial symptoms resulted not so common in patients reacting only to MDA [46].

Moreover, cases of urticaria due to MDI were demonstrated [56–58]. Particularly, Stingeni et al. reported a case of nonatopic man with breathing difficulties for 3 months and urticaria on his face (mala and mandibular areas) for 2 months who worked in a chemical factory manufacturing adhesives and 1 year previously had been assigned to the mixing of polyurethane glues. The symptoms developed a few minutes after every working exposure to the Isonate M143 glue containing diphenylmethane-4,4'-diisocyanate (MDI). This study is the first report of concomitant type I and type IV sensitivities to MDI, as respectively shown by the immediate urticaria-type patch test reaction to Isonate M143, positive radioallergosorbent test to MDI, and delayed positive patch test to MDI and Isonate M143 serial dilutions. Contact urticaria belongs to the class of immediate skin immune response, as also proved by specific IgE antibodies against MDI detected in the patient.

10.3.2   Neurotoxicity

Limited number of studies suggests potential neurotoxic effects from exposures to isocyanates; acute exposure to high levels of TDI vapor has been associated with lightheadedness, headache, insomnia, mental aberrations, impaired gait, loss of consciousness, and coma, while chronic exposures have been associated with alterations in the central and peripheral nervous systems.

One of the first case reports, conducted in 1987, described the accidental exposure of three wharf workers at TDI during an accidental chemical spill. Compared with 2 months postexposure, at 16 months postexposure, Full Scale Intelligence Quotient (IQ) dropped an average of 23 points. Results from additional neuropsychological testing at 16 months postexposure indicated severe deficits in all three subjects in memory, manual dexterity, visuomotor tracking, mental flexibility, ability to detect figure-ground relationships, and word fluency [59].

Reyde et al. reported results of neuropsychological functioning of five men suffering alleged physical, cognitive, and behavioral changes following exposure to MDI. All workers reported experiencing subjective symptoms consisting of respiratory distress, headaches, depression, irritability, decreased calculating ability, and reduced concentration. Wechsler Adult Intelligence Scale-Revised IQ revealed in four of the five subjects weakness on the digit symbol subtest and in attention-concentration testing. The authors concluded that neuropsychological test data support the presence of behavioral and cognitive correlates of CNS injury following exposure to MDI [60].

Recently, Moshe et al. described a case report of a 60-year-old Israeli painter/artist with central and peripheral neuropathic findings. His work was unusual in that he painted large posters with different mixtures of organic solvents, including toluene, xylene, benzene, methyl ethyl ketone, TDI, acetone, and thinner. He did not use any protective gloves and did not wear a mask. After 30 years as a painter, he developed weakness and paresthesia of the hands and feet, intention tremor, and difficulty concentrating with memory deficits. He had mild atrophy and distal weakness of both upper and lower limbs and demonstrated bradykinesia. He was evaluated with several methods and was diagnosed as having peripheral and central neuropathy, including ototoxic hearing loss because of long exposures to organic solvents [61].

In recent years, a systematic review conducted by Hughes et al. demonstrated a lack of quality epidemiological studies in the literature on neurotoxic health effects and exposure to diisocyanates. The available evidence consists mostly of case reports and case series, some of which are listed above. Using the Hill criteria or considerations for causality, the authors found limited evidence for strength of association and consistency [30].

Thus, no robust and confirmed evidence of any primary peripheral or central nervous system neurotoxic effect from diisocyanates has been reported in experimental animal studies. Two-year inhalation studies on both MDI and TDI have been conducted, in which daily observations of clinical signs were made. There were no reports of clinical signs indicative of neurotoxicity [62, 63]. In short-term investigatory studies conducted at higher exposure concentrations than the chronic studies, clinical signs related to respiratory irritation were reported with no indications of neurotoxic effects of MDI or TDI [64–66]. Finally, one sub-chronic study with HDI included a neurobehavioral testing segment, which was negative for such effects [67]. Overall, the animal toxicology test data give no indication of neurotoxic effects from diisocyanates.

10.3.3   Cancerogenesis

As well as to the neurotoxic effects, the carcinogenic risk of TDI and MDI exposure remains an unanswered question.

TDI is classified as a Group 2B carcinogen (possibly carcinogenic to humans) by the IARC [31], as a Category 2 carcinogen (suspect human carcinogen) in the European Commission [68] [68], as reasonably anticipated to be a human carcinogen by the US National Toxicology Program (NTP) [69], and as an A4 carcinogen (not classifiable as a human carcinogen) by ACGIH [32]. These classifications are based on the increased tumor incidences observed by the NTP [70] when TDI in corn oil was administered directly into the stomach of rodents by oral gavage [70]. Oral administration of commercial-grade TDI (analyzed as 85 % 2,4 isomer and 15 % 2,6 isomer) by stomach tube caused hepatocellular adenoma in female rats and mice, fibroadenoma of the mammary gland and islet-cell adenoma of the pancreas in female rats, and acinar-cell adenoma of the pancreas in male rats, while no treatment-related tumors were observed after inhalation exposure of rats and mice. However, this study was flawed both technically (i.e., mishandling of the test material) and conceptually (i.e., gavage exposures) resulting in the formation of toluene diamine, a known animal carcinogen, both prior to and after TDI administration [35].

A long-term inhalation study with TDI was carried out by the International Isocyanate Institute in Sprague-Dawley CD rats and CD-1 mice; in this study, groups of male and female rats and mice were exposed to 0.05 and 0.15 ppm of TDI by inhalation for 6 h/day, 5 days/week for 2 years. Authors concluded that type and incidence of tumors and the number of tumor-bearing animals of either species did not indicate any carcinogenic effect [63]. However, this study was considered inadequate for the evaluation of TDI carcinogenicity by the WHO. The major criticism was that the TDI concentrations used were of magnitudes below acute LC50 values for rats and mice [33, 71]

Regarding MDI, IARC has considered that there is limited evidence in experimental animals for the carcinogenicity of a mixture of monomeric and polymeric MDI. Industrial preparation of MDI was not classifiable as to its carcinogenicity to humans (Group 3) [72].

Experimental studies on rats exposed to MDI by the inhalation route showed that the exposure to polymeric MDI aerosol (a mixture containing 47 % monomeric

MDI and 53 % polymeric MDI) induces severe olfactory epithelium degeneration in females and male Wistar rats at the highest concentration used; at the highest dosage, pulmonary adenomas were observed in males (6/60) and females (2/59) and a pulmonary adenocarcinoma in males (1/60) [62]

In contrast to the study of Reuzel et al. in a long-term carcinogenicity study conducted in female Wistar rats exposed by inhalation to MDI in aerosol form to 0.23, 0.70, and 2.06 mg/m^3-), only 1 of 80 animals of the high-exposure group exhibited a bronchoalveolar adenoma [73].

The carcinogenic risk of TDI and MDI exposure remains an unanswered question. TDI was considered a possible human carcinogen, based on the sufficient evidence of carcinogenicity in animals after oral administration; however, workers are primarily exposed to TDI via inhalation, and it is important to note that toxicity spectrum of TDI metabolites is likely to differ between the routes of administration.

Many studies concluded that no risk could be associated with the inhalation of TDI. Doe and Hoffman assessed the carcinogenic risk of TDI for humans by extrapolating data from the experimental studies in rats and mice and calculating cancer potency. The study concluded that no risk could be associated with the inhalation of TDI [74]. Some epidemiological studies with updates representing the combined long-term mortality experience of more than 17,000 polyurethane foam production workers failed to find an association between occupational exposure to diisocyanates and an increased risk of cancer [75–80]. According to Bolognesi et al., the available human evidence and the experimental data are inadequate to evaluate the carcinogenic risk of isocyanates for humans [33].

Considering the wide range of uses of these compounds and the high number of people occupationally exposed, further experimental and epidemiological investigations on the carcinogenicity of TDI and MDI are urgently needed.

10.4   Conclusion

Isocyanate exposures are common in today's workplace and can cause sensitization and asthma representing an important health risk to workers. Moreover, there is still limited and conflicting knowledge about neurotoxic and carcinogenic effects. Respiratory exposure to isocyanates has long been considered the primary way of exposure. However, respiratory exposures have been reduced through improved hygiene controls and the use of less-volatile isocyanates, thus potentially increasing the relative importance of skin exposure. Despite substantial research on isocyanates, the pathogenic mechanisms, host susceptibility factors, and dose-response relationships remain unclear. Further clinical, epidemiological, and animal research is needed to better understand isocyanate exposure risk factors and elucidate disease mechanism, whereby, preventing worker's exposure to isocyanates represents a critical step in eliminating the health hazards associated with isocyanates. Applying engineering controls, such as closed systems or mechanical ventilation, and requiring personal protective equipment can help limit worker exposure to isocyanates. The use of chemical-resistant clothing and gloves is essential to protecting worker's skin from having contact with isocyanates, and specific types of personal protective equipment (PPE) should be selected according to the hazard assessment results of each workplace.

References

1. Bello D, Woskie SR, Streicher RP, Liu Y, Stowe MH, Eisen EA, et al. Polyisocyanates in occupational environments: a critical review of exposure limits and metrics. Am J Ind Med. 2004;46:480–91.
2. Morgan CJ, Haworth AE. Allergic contact dermatitis from 1,6-hexamethylene diisocyanate in a domestic setting. Contact Dermatitis. 2003;48:224.
3. Deschamps F, Prevost A, Lavaud F, Kochman S. Mechanisms of occupational asthma induced by isocyanates. Ann Occup Hyg. 1998;42:33–6.
4. Redlich CA, Cain H, Wisnewski AV. The immunology and prevention of isocyanate asthma: a model for low molecular weight asthma. Semin Resp Crit Care Med. 1999;20:591–9.
5. Liu Q, Wisnewski AV. Recent developments in diisocyanate asthma. Ann Allergy Asthma Immunol. 2003;90(5Suppl 2):35–41.
6. Day B, Jin R, Basalyga D, Kramarik JA, Karol MH. Formation, solvolysis, and transcarbamoylation reactions of bis(S-glutathionyl) adducts of 2,4- and 2,6-diisocyanatotoluene. Chem Resp Toxicol. 1997;10:424–31.
7. Lange RW, Day BW, Lemus R, Tyurin VA, Kagan VE, Karol MH. Intracellular S-glutathionyl adducts in murine lung and human bronchoepithelial cells after exposure to diisocyanatotoluene. Chem Resp Toxicol. 1999;12:931–6.
8. Sepai O, Henschler D, Sabbioni G. Albumin adducts, hemoglobin adducts, and urinary metabolites in workers exposed to 4,4′-methylenediphenyl diisocyanate. Carcinogenesis. 1995;16:2583–7.
9. Wisnewski AV, Lemus R, Carol MH, Redlich CA. Isocyanate-conjugated human lung epithelial cell proteins: a link between exposure and asthma? J Allergy Clin Immunol. 1999;104:341–7.
10. Lange RW, Lantz RC, Slotz DB, Watkins SC, Sundareshan P, Lemus R, Karol MH. Toluene diisocyanate colocalizes with tubulin on cilia of differentiated human airway epithelial cells. Toxicol Sci. 1999;50:64–71.
11. Wisnewski AV, Srivastava R, Herik C, Xu L, Lemus R, Cain H, et al. Identification of human lung and skin proteins conjugated with hexamethylene diisocyanate *in vitro* and *in vivo*. Am J Resp Crit Care Med. 2000;162:2330–6.
12. Redlich CA, Herrick CA. Lung/skin connections in occupational lung disease. Curr Open Allergy Clin Immunol. 2008;8(2):115–9.
13. NOSH. NOSH health hazard evaluation report. HEAT-99-0196-2860. Naples: Future Aviation; 1999. Cincinnati: National Institute for occupational Safety and Health. Available: http://0-www.cdc.gov.mill1.sjlibrary.org/niosh/hhe/reports/pdfs/1999-0196-2860.pdf. Accessed 12 Jan 2007.
14. Liu Y, Sparer J, Woskie SR, Cullen MR, Chung JS, Holm CT, et al. Qualitative assessment of isocyanate skin exposure in auto body shops: a pilot study. Am J Ind Med. 2000;37(3):265–74.
15. Collin-Hansen I, Stowe M, Ibrahim K, Redlich C, Liu Y, Young's F, et al. Field evaluation of gloves and protective clothing against organic solvents during auto body spray painting (abstract). In: American Industrial Hygiene Association Conference 2006, Chicago. Available: http://www.aiha.org/abs06/po119.htm.

16. Bello D, Herrick CA, Smith TJ, Worskie SR, Streicher RP, Cullen MR, et al. Skin exposure to isocyanates: reasons for concern. Environ Health Perspex. 2007;115:328–35.
17. Swierczynska-Machura D, Palczynski C. Selected patho genetic and clinical aspects of asthma from occupational exposure to diisocyanates. Med Pr. 2012;63(1):97–103. Polish.
18. Bernstein DI, Korbee L, Stauder T, Bernstein JA, Scinto J, Herd ZL, et al. The low prevalence of occupational asthma and antibody-dependent sensitization to diphenylmethanediisocyanate in a plant engineered for minimal exposure to diisocyanates. J Allergy Clin Immunol. 1993;92(3):387–96.
19. Lenaerts-Langanke H. Isocyanate-induced respiratory disease in coal miners. Zel Arbeitsmedizin. 1992;42:2–25.
20. Liss GM, Bernstein DI, Moller DR, Gallagher JS, Stephenson RL, Bernstein IL. Pulmonary and immunologic evaluation of foundry workers exposed to methylene diphenyl diisocyanate (MDI). J Allergy Clin Immunol. 1988;82(1):55–61.
21. Nemery B, Lenaerts L. Exposure to methylene diphenyl diisocyanate in coal mines. Lancet. 1993;341(8840):318.
22. Zammit-Tabona M, Sherkin M, Kijek K, Chan H, Chan-Yeung M. Asthma caused by diphenylmethanediisocyanate in foundry workers. Clinical, bronchial provocation, and immunologic studies. Am Rev Respir Dis. 1983;128(2):226–30.
23. NIOSH. A summary of health hazard evaluations: issues related to occupational exposure to isocyanates, 1989 to 2002. Department of Health and Human Services, Centers for Disease Control and Prevention, National Institute for Occupational Safety and Health. Jan 2004. Available from: http://www.cdc.gov/niosh/docs/2004-116/pdfs/2004-116.pdf.
24. Goossens A, Detienne T, Bruze M. Occupational allergic contact dermatitis caused by isocyanates. Contact Dermatitis. 2002;47(5):304–8.
25. Herrick C, Xu L, Wisnewski AV, Das J, Redlich CA, Bottomly K. A novel mouse model of diisocyanate-induced asthma showing allergic-type inflammation in the lung after inhaled antigen challenge. J Allergy Clin Immunol. 2002;109(5):873–8.
26. Alomar A. Contact dermatitis from a fashion watch. Contact Dermatitis. 1986;15:44–5.
27. Frick M, Bjorkner B, Hamnerius N, Zimerson E. Allergic contact dermatitis from dicyclohexylmethane-4,4′-diisocyanate. Contact Dermatitis. 2003;48(6):305–9.
28. Wilkinson SM, Cartwright PH, Armitage J, English JS. Allergic contact dermatitis from 1,6-diisocyanatohexane in an anti-pill finish. Contact Dermatitis. 1991;25(2):94–6.
29. Frick M, Zimerson E, Karlsson D, Marand A, Skarping G, Isaksson M, et al. Poor correlation between stated and found concentrations of diphenylmethane-4,4′-diisocyanate (4,4′-MDI) in petrolatum patch-test preparations. Contact Dermatitis. 2004;51(2):73–8.
30. Hughes MA, Carson M, Collins MA, Jolly AT, Molenaar DM, Steffens W, Swaen GMH. Does diisocyanate exposure result in neurotoxicity? Clin Toxicol (Phila). 2014;52(4):242–57.
31. IARC. IARC monographs on the evaluation of carcinogenic risks to humans, vol. 71, part 3. Re-evaluation of some organic chemicals, hydrazine and hydrogen peroxide. Lyon: International Agency for Research on Cancer; 1999.
32. ACGIH. 2010 TLVs and BEIs: based on the documentation of the threshold limit values for chemical substances and physical agents and biological exposure indices' American Conference of Governmental Industrial Hygienists, Cincinnati. 2010.
33. Bolognesi C, Baur X, Marczynski B, Norppa H, Sepai O, Sabbioni G. Carcinogenic risk of toluene diisocyanate and 4,4′-methylenediphenyl diisocyanate: epidemiological and experimental evidence. Crit Rev Toxicol. 2001;31(6):737–72.
34. Woolhiser MR, Hayes BB, Meade BJ. A combined murine local lymph node and irritancy assay to predict sensitization and irritancy potential of chemicals. Toxicology. 1998;8(4):245–56.
35. Arnold SM, Collins MA, Graham C, Jolly AT, Parod RJ, Poole A, et al. Risk assessment for consumer exposure to toluene diisocyanates (TDI) derived from polyurethane flexible foam. Regul Toxicol Pharm. 2012;64:504–15.

36. Militello G, Sasseville D, Ditre C, Brod B. Allergic contact dermatitis from isocyanates among sculptors. Dermatitis. 2004;15:150–3.
37. Lidén C. Allergic contact dermatitis from 4,4′-diisocyanto-diphenyl methane (MDI) in a molder. Contact Dermatitis. 1980;6:301.
38. Emmett EA. Allergic contact dermatitis in polyurethane plastic moulders. J Occup Med. 1976;18(12):802–4.
39. White IR, Stewart JR, Rycroft RJ. Allergic contact dermatitis from an organic diisocyanate. Contact Dermatitis. 1983;9(4):300–3.
40. Frick M, Isaksson M, Bjorkner B, Hindsen M, Ponten A, Bruze M. Occupational allergic contact dermatitis in a company manufacturing boards coated with isocyanate lacquer. Contact Dermatitis. 2003;48(5):255–60.
41. Hannu T, Estlander T, Jolanki R. Allergic contact dermatitis due to MDI and MDA from accidental occupational exposure. Contact Dermatitis. 2005;52(2):108–9.
42. Schroder C, Uter W, Schwanitz HJ. Occupational allergic contact dermatitis, partly airborne, due to isocyanates and epoxy resin. Contact Dermatitis. 1999;41(2):117–8.
43. Estlander T, Keskinen H, Jolanki R, Kanerva L. Occupational dermatitis from exposure to polyurethane chemicals. Contact Dermatitis. 1992;27(3):161–5.
44. Tait CP, Delaney TA. Reactions causing reactions: allergic contact dermatitis to an isocyanate metabolite but not to the parent compound. Australas J Dermatol. 1999;40(2):116–7.
45. Kerre S. Allergic contact dermatitis to DMDI in an office application. Contact Dermatitis. 2008;58:313.
46. Aalto-Korte K, Suuronen K, Kuuliala O, Henriks-Eckerman M-L, Jolanki R. Occupational contact allergy to monomeric isocyanates. Contact Dermatitis. 2012;67(2):78–88.
47. Kiec-Swierczynska M, Swierczynska-Machura D, Chomiczewska-Skora D, Nowakowska-Swirta E, Krecisz B. Occupational allergic and irritant contact dermatitis in workers exposed to polyurethane foam. IJOMEH. 2014;27(2):196–205.
48. Vilaplana J, Romaguera C, Grimalt F. Allergic contact dermatitis from aliphatic isocyanate on spectacle frames. Contact Dermatitis. 1987;16:113.
49. Abdalla HI, Balsara RK, O'Riordan AC. Pacemaker contact sensitivity: clinical recognition and management. Ann Thorac Surg. 1994;57:1017–8.
50. Nguyen R, Lee A. Allergic contact dermatitis caused by isocyanates in resin jewellery. Contact Dermatitis. 2012;67:56–7.
51. Aalto-Korte K, Pesonen M, Kuuliala O, Alanko K, Jolanki R. Contact allergy to aliphatic polyisocyanates based on hexamethylene-1,6-diisocyanate (HDI). Contact Dermatitis. 2010;63(6):357–63.
52. Thompson T, Belsito DV. Allergic contact dermatitis from a diisocyanate in wool processing. Contact Dermatitis. 1997;37(5):239.
53. Donovan JCH, Kudla I, DeKoven JG. Rapid development of allergic contact dermatitis from dicyclohexylmethane-4,4′-diisocyanate. Dermatitis. 2009;20(4):214–7.
54. Kanerva L, Tarvainen K, Pinola A, Leino T, Grandlund H, Estlander T, Jolanki R, Forstrom L. A single accidental exposure may result in a chemical burn, primary sensitization and allergic contact dermatitis. Contact Dermatitis. 1994;31:229–35.
55. Liippo J, Lammintausta K. Contact sensitization to 4,4′-diaminodiphenyl methane and to isocyanates among general dermatology patients. Contact Dermatitis. 2008;59:109–14.
56. Kanerva L, Grenquist-Norden B, Piirila P. Occupational IgE-mediated contact urticaria from diphenylmethane-4,4′-diisocyanate (MDI). Contact Dermatitis. 1999;41(1):50.
57. Valks R, Conde-Salazar L, Lopez Barrantes O. Occupational allergic contact urticaria and asthma from diphenylmethane-4,4′-diisocyanate. Contact Dermatitis. 2003;49(3):166–7.
58. Stingeni L, Bellini V, Lisi P. Occupational airborne contact urticaria and asthma: simultaneous immediate and delayed allergy to diphenylmethane-4,4′-diisocyanate. Contact Dermatitis. 2008;58(2):112–3.
59. Singer R, Scott NE. Progression of neuropsychological deficits following toluene diisocyanate exposure. Arch Clin Neuropsychol. 1987;2(2):135–44.

60. Reidy TJ, Bolter JF. Neuropsychological toxicology of methylene diphenyl diisocyanate: a report of five cases. Brain Inj. 1994;8:285–94.
61. Moshe S, Bitchatchi E, Goshen J, Attias J. Neuropathy in an artist exposed to organic solvents in paints: a case study. Arch Environ Health. 2002;57:127–9.
62. Reuzel PG, Arts JH, Lomax LG, Kuijpers MH, Kuper CF, Gembardt C, et al. Chronic inhalation toxicity and carcinogenicity study of respirable polymeric methylene diphenyl diisocyanate (polymeric MDI) aerosol in rats. Fundam Appl Toxicol. 1994;22:195–210.
63. Loeser E. Long-term toxicity and carcinogenicity studies with 2,4/2,6 toluene-diisocyanate (80/20) in rats and mice. Toxicol Lett. 1983;15:71–81.
64. Pauluhn J. Comparative analysis of pulmonary irritation by measurements of Penh and protein in bronchoalveolar lavage fluid in brown Norway rats and Wistar rats exposed to irritant aerosols. Inhal Toxicol. 2004;16:159–75.
65. Reuzel PG, Kuper CF, Feron VJ, Appelman LM, Loser E. Acute, subacute, and subchronic inhalation toxicity studies of respirable polymeric methylene diphenyl diisocyanate (polymeric MDI) aerosol in rats. Fundam Appl Toxicol. 1994;22:186–94.
66. Johnson VJ, Yucesoy B, Reynolds JS, Fluharty K, Wang W, Richardson D, Luster MI. Inhalation of toluene diisocyanate vapor induces allergic rhinitis in mice. J Immunol. 2007;79:1864–71.
67. Astroff AB, Sheets LP, Sturdivant DW, Stuart BP, Shiotsuka RN, Simon GS, et al. A combined reproduction, neonatal development, and neurotoxicity study with 1,6-hexamethylene diisocyanate (HDI) in the rat. Reprod Toxicol. 2000;14:135–46.
68. European Commission. Commission Directive 98/98/EC of 15 December 1998 adapting to technical progress for the 25 time Council Directive 67/548/EEC on the approximation of laws, regulations and administrative provisions relating to the classification, packaging and labelling of dangerous substances. Off J Eur Commun. 1998;41(L355):386–9.
69. NTP. Report on carcinogens, 12th ed. US Department of Health and Human Services, Public Health Service, National Toxicology Program. 2011.
70. NTP. Toxicology and carcinogenesis studies of commercial grade 2,4(80%)- and 2,6(20%)-toluene diisocyanate in F344/N rats and B6C3F1 mice (gavage studies).US Department of Health and Human Services. National Toxicology Program. NTP TR 251; NIH Publication No. 86-2507. Research Triangle Park, NC. 1986.
71. WHO World Health Organization. Environmental health criteria 75, toluene diisocyanate. Geneva: WHO; 1987.
72. IARC. 4,4′-methylenediphenyl diisocyanate and polymeric4,4′-methylenediphenyl diisocyanate. IARC Monogr Eval Carcinog Risks Chem Hum. 1999;71:1049–58.
73. Hoymann, et al. 1995 (unpublished study) in: EPA 1998. Available at: http://www.epa.gov.
74. Doe JE, Hoffman HD. Toluene diisocyanate: an assessment of carcinogenic risk following oral and inhalation exposure. Toxicol Ind Health. 1990;6:599–621.
75. Hagmar L, Welinder H, Mikoczy Z. Cancer incidence and mortality in the Swedish polyurethane foam manufacturing industry. Br J Ind Med. 1993;50:537–43.
76. Hagmar L, Stroemberg U, Welinder H, Mikoczy Z. Incidence of cancer and exposure to toluene diisocyanate and methylene diphenyl diisocyanate: a cohort based case-referent study in the polyurethane foam manufacturing industry. Br J Ind Med. 1993;50:1003–7.
77. Mikoczy Z, Welinder H, Tinnerberg H, Hagmar L. Cancer incidence and mortality of isocyanate exposed workers from the Swedish polyurethane foam industry: updated findings 1959–98. Occup Environ Med. 2004;61(5):432–7.
78. Schnorr TM, Steenland K, Egeland GM, Boeniger M, Egilman D. Mortality of workers exposed to toluene diisocyanate in the polyurethane foam industry. Occup Environ Med. 1996;53(10):703–7.
79. Sorahan T, Nichols L. Mortality and cancer morbidity of production workers in the UK flexible polyurethane foam industry: updated findings 1958–98. Occup Environ Med. 2002;59(11):751–8.
80. Sorahan T, Pope D. Mortality and cancer morbidity of production workers in the United Kingdom flexible polyurethane foam industry. Br J Ind Med. 1993;50:528–36.

Chapter 11
Skin Exposure to Nanoparticles and Possible Sensitization Risk

Francesca Larese Filon

Abstract Due to the increased production and use of nanoparticles (NPs), there are workers and consumers that can be exposed to NPs. There is a debate among scientists to define possible effects related to this exposure and there are more open questions. The review evaluates the recent knowledge on this topic trying to classify NPs in relation to their hazard for skin exposure, both for workers and consumers. While the same kind of NPs can be safe for skin contact (such as titanium dioxide and zinc oxide), others can exert a sensitization effect such as NPs that can release sensitizing metals (i.e., Ni, Pd, Co), as well as a toxic effects for NPs that can release toxic metals such as Cd or As.

Due to the high surface/mass ratio, NPs can release more metals than bulk materials, increasing the risk of skin or systemic effects after the skin contact with them. Moreover, NP size and the impairment of the skin barrier of exposed workers and consumers are crucial points to be evaluated because they both can contribute to NPs exposure and skin absorption.

Labeling is needed for NPs and products containing sensitizing or toxic metals to advise users to protect them from direct contact with the skin.

Keywords Nanoparticles • Skin exposure • Skin absorption • Allergic sensitization

11.1 Introduction

Engineered NPs production is growing in quantity for industrial application [1]. The National Science Foundation has estimated that by 2020, nanotechnology will employ six million workers [2, 3]. Moreover, many workers and consumers are handling nano-embedded products that are already available on the market. Many

F. Larese Filon (✉)
Unit of Occupational Medicine, Department of Medical Sciences, University of Trieste,
Via della Pietà 19, 34129 Trieste, Italy
e-mail: larese@units.it

© Springer Science+Business Media Singapore 2017
T. Otsuki et al. (eds.), *Allergy and Immunotoxicology in Occupational Health*,
Current Topics in Environmental Health and Preventive Medicine,
DOI 10.1007/978-981-10-0351-6_11

cosmetics contain NPs, mainly titanium dioxide and zinc oxide, due to the better properties of creams. Many textiles, wound dressings, deodorants, antiperspirants, pigments, varnishes, electronic devices, catalytic converters, and fuel cells are prepared using NPs and can release NPs during their use. NPs can be released from nano-enabled products, such as pastes, paints, glues, etc. and are potential sources of dermal exposure to NPs [4–7].

NPs may exhibit new physicochemical properties due to the small size (1–100 nm) with a faster and more efficient penetration into the human body than bulk materials. Their high surface/mass ratio can cause a higher release of toxic substances compared to non-nanopowders.

Many studies have demonstrated the safe profile of NPs used in cosmetics [8, 9], and the widespread use without any reported adverse effect can confirm that these kinds of NPs did not harm the skin or the body. Different questions arise for other NPs that are present in objects or other products that can have a possible local effect or can penetrate the skin barrier with local or systemic effects [10–12]. As different NPs cannot be considered in the same way, we need to evaluate different classes of NPs to define their hazard related to skin contact [12]. Data are scanty on human/worker exposure, but recently a worker exposed to nano-nickel developed contact dermatitis and occupational asthma [13] handling nanoscale nickel NPs without protection measures that are already suggested for workers exposed to NPs [1, 2]. She worked with nanoscale nickel without a local exhaustion system nor in a glove box, and she did not wear a respiratory mask that can protect exposed workers [14, 15]. Nanosized metallic nickel (Ni) has special properties, i.e., high surface energy, high magnetism, and high surface area which makes it ideal for a number of industrial processes [16]. There are some data to indicate that nanosized metallic nickel (20 nm) is more toxic than standard-sized nickel (5 mm) in a rat model of lung toxicity [17]. Crosera et al. [18] evaluate nickel NP skin absorption through human skin using an ex vivo approach finding that these NPs applied on skin surface cause an increase of nickel content into the skin and a significant permeation flux through the skin, higher when a damaged skin protocol was used. They stated that preventive measures are needed when NiNPs are produced and used due to their higher potential to enter in our body compared to bulk nickel.

Moreover, it is advisable to implement surveillance as NP and nano-embedded products become more pervasive in the workplace [19–21].

The aim of this review is to evaluate available literature on skin exposure to NP to define aspects to be considered for risk assessment, with special attention for NPs containing sensitizing metals.

11.2   Material and Methods

Literature were evaluated using the terms "NP skin exposure," "nanomaterial skin exposure," "irritant contact dermatitis epidemiology," and "allergic contact dermatitis epidemiology" in PubMed, Thomson Reuters Web of Science, and Scopus databases. Governmental institution guidelines (NIOSH) were used to insure a practical approach to workers' protection. A total of 293 were selected and 54 were used to elaborate this review.

11.3 Results

11.3.1 When Skin Exposure to NPs Is Possible?

People can be exposed intentionally, because they apply on the skin products that contain NPs, such as creams, cosmetics, and wound dressing. Others can wear textile embedded with silver NPs or they touch objects coated with nano-products. Workers can be exposed non-intentionally because they are producing, using, manufacturing, handling, and processing NPs or products that can release NPs. Also during the use of products containing NPs, it is possible a release from objects, varnishes, glues, or other products that contain NPs. Since it is not compulsory the labeling of products containing NPs, there are many commercially available products that are made using also NPs and that can come in contact with the skin. The European Agency for Safety and Health at Work reported that the biggest risk of exposure to NPs were in construction, health care, energy conversion and use, automobile (and aerospace) industry, chemical industry, and electronics and communication [22]. Table 11.1 reports a non-exhaustive list of industries/products.

11.3.2 Relevant Aspects for Skin Exposure to NPs

11.3.2.1 Source Domains

Dermal exposure can be evaluated using the conceptual framework elaborated by Schneider et al. [23]. The source of contamination is NPs produced or released from objects. From the source domains, the NPs can deposit on the skin or on other surfaces (*direct contact*). NPs can be transported to the air zone, and from there they can contaminate the skin and surfaces by *deposition*. Protective gloves and aprons can be contaminated themselves and resuspension of NPs can happen. Finally NPs can be *transferred* to other surfaces and to the perioral region causing *inadvertent intake and ingestion*. More information on risk resulting from **skin** contact can be found in BauA [24].

Van Duuren-Stuurman et al. in 2008 [25] studied dermal exposure to NPs in ten European enterprises using an observation model (Dermal Exposure Assessment, DREAM). In the majority of tasks observed (39/45), dermal exposure cannot be excluded, and the main routes for exposure were transfer and direct contact.

Table 11.1 Examples of industries where skin exposure to NPs is possible (non-exhaustive)

Industries	Material handled	Potential for skin exposure
Production of nanomaterials	NPs	Yes
Production of nanocomposites	NPs	Yes
Pharmaceutical industry	NPs, liquid	Yes
Toner production	NPs	Yes
Food production	Liquid	Yes
Tattoo ink production and application	NPs	Yes also inside the skin
Plant protection fertilizers	Liquids	Yes
Production and use of concrete	Powders	Yes
Paint production	Liquid and powders	Yes
Ink production	Liquid	Yes
Cosmetics production	Powders	Yes
Coating application in textiles, plastics, cleaning, health care, homecare	Liquid, powders	Yes
Electronic production	Liquid, powders	Yes
Battery production	Liquid, powders	Yes
Black rubber production	Powders	Yes
Sport industry	Powders	Yes
Fuel production	Liquid	Yes
Waste treatments	All	Yes

11.3.2.2 NP Characteristics

NPs emitted from processes or released from objects or textiles agglomerate and settle on the skin and on surfaces. Therefore, in general, the skin comes in contact with agglomerated NPs with a diameter bigger than 100 nm, and the presence of acid pH and sweat can increase their tendency to aggregate. Moreover, in contact with sweat, NPs can release metals or impurities in higher amount than bulk material for the high ratio surface/mass. These aspects are more relevant when toxic or sensitized metals can be released (Cd, Ni, Pd, Ag, etc.) [12].

11.3.2.3 Size

Larese Filon et al. in [12] suggested some critical sizes to evaluate NP skin hazard: for NPs <4 nm, penetration has been demonstrated; for NPs 4–20 nm, skin penetration/permeation is possible, probably through follicles; for NPs 21–45 nm, skin absorption can be possible only on impaired skin; and for NPs >45 nm, skin absorption is unlikely in healthy skin.

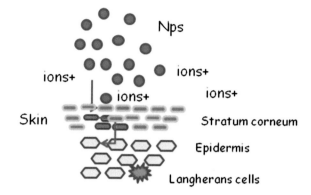

Fig. 11.1 Metal NPs can release more ions than bulk metals and skin absorption can happen as ions or as NPs

11.3.2.4 Release of Toxic or Sensitization Substances

Due to their high surface/mass ratio, NPs can release metals in ionic form that can penetrate the skin inducing local or systemic effects. NPs can induce in more efficient way skin sensitization with respect to bulk materials. Ni, Cd, Co, and Pd NPs can release metals that can cause allergic contact dermatitis (Fig. 11.1). Journey and Goldman reported in 2014 [13] a case of skin and respiratory sensitization in women exposed to NiNPs. No other case reports are available in literature.

Quantum dots containing Cd can be absorbed through the skin reaching general blood circulation causing sign of systemic intoxication of Cd in exposed animals [26], while no data are available in exposed workers. Polycyclic aromatic hydrocarbons can be released from NPs [27], and their carcinogen effect could be exerted on the skin. Therefore, no human data are available on that.

11.3.2.5 Coating and pH

Very few data are available on this topic, but coating and pH could influence dissolution, release of sensitized or toxic metals, and also persistence on the skin. While many data are available on different cells in vitro, no data are available on real work scenario. Ovissipour et al. [28] studied decontamination of tomatoes treated with different NPs, and he found that decontamination could be difficult from surfaces in particular conditions of pH of the solution used and isoelectric point of NPs.

11.3.3 Skin Contamination

11.3.3.1 Area of the Skin Contaminated with NPs

Absorption of NPs through the skin is a function of surface area contaminated, applied dose, time of contact, thickness of the membrane, and characteristics of the NPs, On the other site, the use of protective measures to avoid skin contamination is extremely important, due to the difficulties in removal of NPs from the skin.

11.3.3.2   Applied Dose

The amount of NPs that come in contact to the skin is important for decontamination purposes and for the loading on the skin surface. Nevertheless, in the condition of substances with very low permeation rate, such as NPs, the dose could be not relevant because a decontamination is not easy or possible, and NPs can be stored in hair follicles and from there they can release ions. Moreover, NPs can penetrate and permeate the skin if their size is less than 45 nm, as suggested by Larese Filon et al. [12].

11.3.3.3   Time of Contact

Skin effect or absorption can be more effective when skin is exposed for longer period. One of the crucial aspects is that after contact with NPs, it is quite difficult to clean the skin because NPs are very adhesive to the skin and they reach the hair follicles where they cannot be removed. In this condition also, after a short contact with the skin, NPs cannot be removed by the cleaning procedures. There are no, in our knowledge, studies on this topic, but there are experimental data that demonstrated that hair follicles are the "storage" place for NPs that can come in contact to the skin [29]. Moreover, one study evaluated the cleaning effect on tomatoes contaminated by NPs washed using deionized water. The washing was effective to remove alumina NPs but not titania and silica [29]. The NPs persistence on the surface was explained with differences between pH of the washing solution and NPs isoelectric point. The Fourier transform infrared spectroscopy results showed that some NPs can bind to certain biochemical components such as polysaccharides and proteins on the surface of tomato skins.

In human skin, NPs can penetrate between the stratum corneum and inside the hair follicles when NPs are flexible or when rigid NPs are smaller than 40–45 nm, particularly when the skin is impaired [12]. From hair follicles NPs can release toxic or sensitized substances or can cross the epithelia reaching the derma. Rancan et al. [29] demonstrated that silica NPs can reach Langerhans cells after they have been stored in hair follicles.

11.3.3.4   Condition of the Skin Barrier

Occupational skin diseases (OSD) are extremely common in worker populations. The European Agency for Safety and Health at Work, EU-OSHA, EU-25 report 2008 [30], reported that they constitute a top-priority public health problem. The economic burden of OSD in the EU exceeds € 5 billion spent every year on treatment, compensation, and loss of productivity [31]. They represent up to 35 % of all reported occupational diseases [32, 33]. The impairment of the skin is frequent in some professions, particularly in wet workers, construction workers, health-care workers, hairdressers, mechanics, etc. that are doing "wet work" or are in contact with irritants and sensitizing agents.

The impairment of the skin barrier increases the risk of NPs penetration because NPs can reach easily the basal layers of the epidermis and hair follicles [29]. The impairment of the skin increases NPs penetration 4–100 times [34–36], and for some NPs, such as titanium dioxide, skin penetration is possible only in impaired skin [37]. Frequent exposure to water, irritant chemicals, detergents, disinfectants, and powders can lead to fissuring of the skin [38]. Moreover it is possible for the skin barrier to be compromised, although there are no visible signs [39]. In this case, the contamination of the skin with NPs can cause an increased risk of NPs penetration into the skin and possible effects. In vitro data performed using human skin and Franz cells demonstrated that, obviously, the impairment of the skin increases significantly the metal content inside the skin and skin absorption for many metal NPs [18, 34, 36, 40, 41].

11.3.4 Skin Decontamination and Cleansing Procedures

No data are available on the better way to decontaminate and to clean the skin after contact with NPs. The possible persistence of NPs on skin surface, inside the stratum corneum, and the storage on hair follicles suggests the need to avoid direct skin contact with NPs. Decontamination of tomato surface after contact with alumina, silica, and titania NPs can be more or less effective in function of pH of the solution used and the isoelectric point of the NPs [28]. Moreover, cleansing procedures can enhance penetration, increasing pH of the skin and reducing the skin barrier properties. No data are available on workers but data on decontamination from the skin of lead powders (non-nano) in in vitro condition demonstrated that different cleaning procedures can influence decontamination effectiveness and can increase skin absorption of lead [42]. Considering that decontamination procedures can be less effective after the contact with NPs, we stress the need to avoid skin contamination at all.

11.3.5 Skin Protection

Gloves made of neoprene, nitrile, or other chemical-resistant gloves should be used and changed frequently or whenever they are visibly worn, torn, or contaminated to protect the hands from the direct or indirect contact with NPs [1]. We suggest the use of double gloves to increase the protection. Work apron with long trousers, long sleeves, gauntlets, and caps are recommended to avoid contamination with other parts of the body skin that can increase the exposed area and through skin absorption of NPs.

11.4   Discussion and Conclusions

Skin exposure to NPs can be relevant for local or systemic effect in a particular condition and where it is possible skin contact with NPs that can release sensitizing (i.e., Ni, Pd, Co) or toxic metals (i.e., Cd, As). The high rate surface/mass permits NPs to release metallic ions in higher amount *vs* bulk material. Ions can penetrate the skin and cause allergic sensitization or allergic symptoms in already sensitized subjects or can induce allergic sensitization. Moreover, there is only one case report of sensitization and symptoms in a woman exposed to nickel NPs [13], while only animal data are available on cadmium presence into internal organs in rats exposed via skin to Cd-selenite quantum dots [26]. NPs can release polyaromatic hydrocarbons (PAH) that can have local or systemic effects, due also to their carcinogen effect [27].

For NPs that cannot release toxic/sensitizing metals or chemicals, we have two options:

1. Soft NPs as liposomes can penetrate and permeate the skin because they can squeeze between cells.
2. Rigid NPs: only very small NPs can penetrate and permeate the intact skin (<4 nm). For NPs 4–20 nm, a skin penetration/permeation is possible, probably through follicles; for NPs 21–45 nm, skin absorption can be possible only on impaired skin; for NPs >45 nm, skin absorption is unlikely in healthy skin.

   In these conditions, the presence of an impaired skin barrier in workers needs to be evaluated, since skin absorption can happen also for bigger NPs.

Moreover, considering that NPs can persist on the skin despite decontaminate measures, it is compulsory to avoid skin contamination using personal protective equipment. Labeling is needed for NPs and products containing sensitizing or toxic metals to advise users to protect them from direct contact with the skin.

Conflict of Interest None

References

1. NIOSH. General safe practices for working with engineered nanomaterials in research laboratories. Cinncinnati: Department of Health and Human Services, Centers for Disease. Control and Prevention, National Institute for Occupational Safety and Health; 2012.
2. NIOSH Current strategies for engineering controls in nanomaterial production and downstream handling processes. Cincinnati: U.S. Department of Health and Human Services, Centers for Disease Control and Prevention, National Institute for Occupational Safety and Health, DHHS (NIOSH) Publication No. 2014–102.
3. IEEE-USA – Eye on Washington. House subcommittee explores economic benefits of federal nanotechnology initiative. 2011. https://science.house.gov/news/press-releases/subcommittee-explores-economic-benefits-federal-nanotechnology-initiative. Accessed 31 Jan 2016.
4. Aitken RJ, Chaudhry MQ, Boxall ABA, Hull M. Manufacture and use of nanomaterials: current status in the UK and global trends. Occup Med. 2006;56:300–6.
5. Aitken RJ, Creely KS, Tran CL. Nanoparticles: an occupational hygiene review, HSE Research Report 274. London: HSE Books; 2004.

6. Bianco C, Kezic S, Visser MJ, Pluut O, Adami G, Krystek P. Pilot study on the identification of silver in skin layers and urine after dermal exposure to a functionalized textile. Talanta. 2015;136:23–8. doi:10.1016/j.talanta.2014.12.043.

7. Bianco C, Kezic S, Crosera M, Svetličić V, Šegota S, Maina G, Romano C, Larese F, Adami G. *In vitro* percutaneous penetration and characterization of silver from silver-containing textiles. Int J Nanomedicine. 2015;10:1899–908. doi:10.2147/IJN.S78345. eCollection 2015.

8. SCCP – Scientific Committee on Consumer Products. Preliminary opinion on safety of nano-materials in cosmetic products. Brussels: European Commission; 2007. http://ec.europa.eu/health/archive/ph_risk/committees/04_sccp/docs/sccp_o_123.pdf. Accessed 12 Dec 2015.

9. NANODERM Eu project http://www.uni-leipzig.de/~nanoderm/ Project ID:QLK4-CT-2002-02678. Accessed 20 Dec 2015.

10. Crosera M, Bovenzi M, Maina G, Adami G, Zanette C, Florio C, Filon Larese F. Nanoparticle dermal absorption and toxicity: a review of the literature. Int Arch Occup Environ Health. 2009;82:1043–55.

11. Labouta HI, Schneider M. Interaction of inorganic nanoparticles with the skin barrier: current status and critical review. Nanomedicine. 2013;9:39–54.

12. Larese Filon F, Mauro M, Adami G, Bovenzi M, Crosera M. Nanoparticles skin absorption: new aspects for a safety profile evaluation. Reg Toxicol Pharmacol. 2015;72:310–22.

13. Journeay WS, Goldman RH. Occupational handling of nickel nanoparticles: a case report. Am J Ind Med. 2014;57:1073–6.

14. Shaffer RE, Rengasamy S. Respiratory protection against airborne nanoparticles: a review. J Nanopart Res. 2009;11:1661–72.

15. Groso A, Petri-Fink A, Magrez A, Riediker M, Meyer T. Management of nanomaterials safety in research environment. Part Fibre Toxicol. 2010;7:40–3.

16. Zhao J, Shi X, Castranova V, Ding M. Occupational toxicology of nickel and nickel com-pounds. J Environ Pathol Toxicol Oncol. 2009;28:177–208.

17. Zhang Q, Kusaka Y, Zhu X, Sato K, Mo Y, Kluz T, Donaldson K. Comparative toxicity of standard nickel and ultrafine nickel in lung after intratracheal instillation. J Occup Health. 2003;45:23–30.

18. Crosera M, Adami G, Mauro M, Bovenzi M, Baracchini E, Larese Filon F. *In vitro* dermal penetration of nickel nanoparticles. Chemosphere. 2015;145:301–6. doi:10.1016/j.chemosphere.2015.11.076.

19. Dahm MM, Yencken MS, Schubauer-Berigan MK. Exposure control strategies in the carbona-ceous nanomaterial industry. J Occup Environ Med. 2011;53:S68–73.

20. Song J, Quee D, Yu L, Gunaratnam S. Current surveillance plan for persons handling nanoma-terials in the National University of Singapore. J Occup Environ Med. 2011;53(6 Suppl):S25–7.

21. Lee J, Mun J, Park J, Yu I. A health surveillance case study on workers who manufacture silver nanomaterials. Nanotoxicology. 2012;6(6):667–9.

22. Kaluza S, Balderhaar JK, Orthen B, Honnert B, Jankowska E, Pietrowski P, Rosell MG, Tanarro C, Tejedor J, Zugasti A. Workplace exposure to nanoparticles. European Agency for Health and Safety at Work. 2009.

23. Schneider T, Vermeulen R, Brouwer DH, Cherrie JW, Kromhout H, Fogh CL. Conceptual model for assessment of dermal exposure. Occup Environ Med. 1999;56:765–73.

24. Bau A. Risk resulting from skin contact – identification, assessment, measures. 2008. http://www.baua.de/en/Topics-from-A-to-Z/Hazardous-Substances/TRGS/pdf/TRGS-401.pdf%3F__blob=publicationFile%26v=4. Accessed 15 Mar 2016.

25. Van Duuren-Stuurman, Pelzer J, Moehlmann C, Berges M, Bard D, Wake D, Mark D, Janskowska E, Brouwer D. A structured observational method to assess dermal exposure to manufactured nanoparticles DREAM as an initial assessment tool. Int J Occup Environ Health. 2010;16:399–405.

26. Tang L, Zhang C, Song G, Jin X, Xu Z. *In vivo* skin penetration and metabolic path of quantum dots. Sci Chin Life Sci. 2013;56(2):181–8.

27. Plata DL, Gschwend PM, Reddy CM. Industrially synthesized single-walled carbon nano-tubes: compositional data for users, environmental risk assessments, and source apportion-ment. Nanotechnology. 2008;19:185706.

28. Ovissipour M, Sablani SS, Rasco B. Engineered nanoparticle adhesion and removal from tomato surfaces. J Agric Food Chem. 2013;61(42):10183–90. doi:10.1021/jf4018228. Epub 2013 Oct 14.
29. Rancan F, Gao Q, Graf C, Troppens S, Hadam S, Vogt A. Skin penetration and cellular uptake of amorphous silica nanoparticles with variable size, surface functionalization and colloidal stability. ACS Nano. 2012;8:6829–42.
30. European Agency for Safety and Health at Work, EU-OSHA, EU-25 report. Occupational skin diseases and dermal exposure in the European Union. 2008. https://osha.europa.eu/en/node/6875/file_view. Accessed 18 Feb 2106.
31. Sartorelli P, Kezic S, Larese Filon F, John SM. Prevention of occupational dermatitis. Int J Immunopathol Pharmacol. 2011;24(1 Suppl):89S–93.
32. Diepgen TL, Andersen KE, Brandao FM, Bruze M, Bruynzeel DP, Frosch P, Gonçalo M, Goossens A, Le Coz CJ, Rustemeyer T, White IR, Agner T, European Environmental and Contact Dermatitis Research Group. Hand eczema classification: a cross-sectional, multicentre study of the aetiology and morphology of hand eczema. Br J Dermatol. 2009;160:353–8.
33. Keegel T, Moyle M, Dharmage S, Frowen K, Nixon R. The epidemiology of occupational contact dermatitis (1990–2007): a systematic review. Int J Dermatol. 2009;48(6):571–8. doi:10.1111/j.1365-4632.2009.04004.x. Review.
34. Larese Filon F, D'Agostin F, Bovenzi M, Crosera M, Adami G, Romano C, Maina G. Human skin penetration of silver nanoparticles through intact and damaged skin. Toxicology. 2009;255:33–7.
35. Larese Filon F, Crosera M, Adami G, Bovenzi M, Rossi F, Maina G. Human skin penetration of gold nanoparticles through intact and damaged skin. Nanotoxicology. 2011;5:493–501.
36. Crosera M, Prodi A, Mauro M, Pelin M, Florio C, Bellomo F, Adami G, Apostoli P, De Palma G, Bovenzi M, Campanini M, Filon FL. Titanium dioxide nanoparticle penetration into the skin and effects on HaCaT cells. Int J Environ Res Public Health. 2015;12(8):9282–97.
37. Larese Filon F, Crosera M, Timeus E, Adami G, Bovenzi M, Ponti J, Maina G. Human skin penetration of cobalt nanoparticles through intact and damaged skin. Toxicol Vitro. 2013;27:121–7.
38. Chew AL, Maibach HI. Occupational issues of irritant contact dermatitis. Int Arch Occup Environ Health. 2003;76(5):339–46.
39. Kezic S, Visser MJ, Verbeek MM. Individual susceptibility to occupational contact dermatitis. Ind Health. 2009;47:469–78.
40. Mauro M, Crosera M, Bianco C, Adami G, Montini T, Fornasiero P, Bovenzi M, Larese F. Human skin penetration of platinum and rhodium nanoparticles through intact and damaged skin. J Nanoparticles Res. 2015;17:253.
41. Mauro M, Crosera M, Pelin M, Florio C, Bellomo F, Adami G, Apostoli P, De Palma G, Bovenzi M, Campanini M, Filon FL. Cobalt oxide nanoparticles: behavior towards intact and impaired human skin and keratinocytes toxicity. Int J Environ Res Public Health. 2015;12(7):8263–80.
42. Larese Filon F, Boeniger M, Maina G, Adami G, Spinelli P, Damian A. Skin absorption of inorganic lead (PbO) and the effect of skin cleansers. J Occup Environ Med. 2006;84:692–9.

Printed in the United States
By Bookmasters